I0478335

Table of Contents

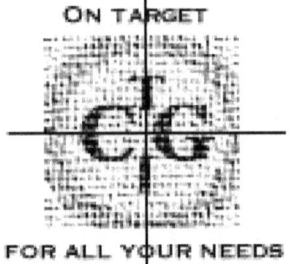

ON TARGET

FOR ALL YOUR NEEDS

THE CANCER GROUP INSTITUTE

23825 Anza Avenue
Suite. #108
Torrance, California – 90505
© 2017
818.491.7738
www.CancerGroup.com

LEUKEMIA
(Acute & Chronic)

Disclaimer

CancerGroup.com serves only as a clearinghouse for medical and health information and does not directly or indirectly practice medicine. Any information provided by *CancerGroup.com* is intended solely for educating our clients and should not be construed as medical advice or guidance, which should always be obtained from a physician or other licensed health care professional. As such, the client assumes full responsibility for the appropriate use of medical information contained in this publication and agrees to hold *CancerGroup.com* and any of its third party providers harmless from any and all claims or actions arising from clients' use or reliance on this publication. Although *CancerGroup.com* makes every reasonable attempt to conduct a thorough search of the published medical literature, the possibility exists that some significant articles may be missed.

What is Leukemia?

Leukemia is a cancer of the blood cells. There are various types of blood cells, red blood cells to carry oxygen and white blood cells to fight infections. Also, another type of blood cell called **"platelets"** are fragments which assist in clotting.

Leukemia is not a single disease, but a group of malignancies in which the bone marrow and other blood-forming organs produce excessive numbers of white blood cells. The extra cells, which are usually immature or abnormal, suppress the production of normal white blood cells, the function of which is to protect the body against infection.

Malignant cells "take over" the bone marrow and prevent it from producing red blood cells, which transport oxygen around the body, and platelets, which help blood clot. They also invade other organs, such as the liver, spleen, lymph nodes, genitals, and brain.

Leukemias are classified by the type of white blood cell that is proliferating abnormally and by how fast the disease is progressing. Acute leukemia can be fatal in weeks or months without aggressive treatment. Chronic leukemia progresses more slowly and may be "indolent"-producing no symptoms-for 20 years or longer.

A patient with leukemia may go to the doctor feeling extremely sick, complaining of recur-rent infections, bleeding, bruising, bone tenderness, fever, chills, sweats, weakness, fatigue, headaches, or swelling in the neck, armpits or groin.

On the other hand, the patient may have no symptoms at all and the disease may be discovered by chance from a routine blood test.

A normal blood smear contains many red cells and platelets and a few white cells. In leukemia, the blood usually contains many abnormal white

Copyright - 2017. Published by Cancer Group Institute. www.cancergroup.com

cells and not enough red cells and platelets. Such an abnormal blood count is the physician's first clue that the patient may have leukemia, but it is not sufficient for a diagnosis.

The next step is a bone marrow aspiration and biopsy. Marrow is withdrawn from the body by suction, using a large needle and a syringe, and microscopically examined. This crucial diagnostic test is followed by more laboratory tests to identify what type of leukemia the patient has. A precise diagnosis is important because different types of disease respond to different therapies.

If the diagnosis is chronic leukemia and the patient has no symptoms, treatment may not be required for months or even years.

Patients with some types of chronic leukemia may be treated with splenectomy, or surgical removal of the spleen. This organ, located behind the stomach, sometimes becomes enlarged after leukemic cells invade it.

Acute Leukemia.

A diagnosis of acute leukemia usually means immediate hospitalization. Patients are given antibiotics, or other appropriate therapy, for infections and other symptoms. Because leukemia patients need frequent transfusions of blood and blood products, they must be treated at medical centers with access to large quantities of such products.

Chemotherapy for acute leukemia involves two phases: an induction phase, in which the patient is aggressively treated with a combination of powerful drugs in an effort to kill all the leukemic cells, and a consolidation phase, using either the same or different drugs, which begins once the disease has gone into remission.

The two main types of acute leukemia are acute lymphocytic leukemia and acute myelogenous leukemia. Currently approved drugs to treat acute lymphocytic leukemia include vincristine (Oncovin), prednisone (Deltasone), asparaginase (Elspar), cyclophosphamide (Cytoxan, Neosar), and cytarabine (Cytosar). Approved drugs for acute myelogenous leukemia include daunorubicin, also called daunomycin (Cerubidine), and cytarabine (Cytosar).

These drugs are cytotoxic, which means they kill not only cancerous cells but also normal cells, particularly in the bone marrow. The patient's immune system-already malfunctioning because of the proliferation of leukemic cells-is completely knocked out, leaving the individual defenseless against bacterial and fungal infections.

New Drugs for Chronic Leukemia.

Most of the recent advances in drug therapy for leukemia involve compounds effective against chronic leukemia, particularly chronic lymphocytic leukemia (CLL), the most common form of adult leukemia in the United States. It is a slowly progressing disease that usually affects people over 50.

Treatment for chronic leukemia is generally less aggressive than for acute leukemia and is often given on an outpatient basis. The current standard therapy for CLL is cyclophosphamide or chlorambucil (Leukeran), sometimes in combination with prednisone (Deltasone) or prednisolone (Hydeltra, Pediapred). While these drugs can relieve symptoms, many patients experience significant side effects and eventually stop responding.

Fludarabine (Fludara) was approved by FDA in April 1991 to treat patients who do not respond to other therapies for CLL. In NCI-sponsored clinical trials involving such patients, 32 to 48 percent responded to fludarabine and 13 percent achieved complete remission.

Researchers think fludarabine works by inhibiting reproduction of abnormal lymphocytes, a type of white blood cell. The drug belongs to a unique class of medications known as purine analogues. Purines are nitrogen-based molecules used as building blocks of DNA, the basic genetic material of living organisms.

Another type of chronic leukemia is chronic myelogenous leukemia (CML). Currently approved drugs for CML are busulfan (Myleran) and hydroxyurea (Hydrea).

In January 1992, FDA approved pentostatin (Nipent) for treating patients with a rare form of chronic leukemia called hairy cell leukemia who do not respond to alpha interferon, the standard therapy. In clinical trials, 70 percent of patients taking pentostatin achieved complete, long-term remission. The drug is a derivative of Streptomyces antibioticus, a fungus from which many antibiotics, including tetracycline, are derived.

An experimental drug, 2CDA, has also shown results against hairy cell leukemia, achieving long-term remissions in 80 to 85 percent of patients treated in clinical trials. This drug is currently available under FDA's Treatment IND regulations. (IND stands for investigational new drug.) Under these regulations, desperately ill patients who do not respond to conventional therapy can receive promising experimental drugs before completion of the review needed for full approval.

The oncologic drug advisory committee recommended that FDA approve 2CDA for the treatment of hairy cell leukemia.

2CDA is an antimetabolite, one of a group of drugs that prevent cell growth by interfering with essential enzyme reactions. A major difference between 2CDA and pentostatin is that a complete course of 2CDA can be given in one week, while treatment with pentostatin extends over a six-month period.

Fludara, Nipent and 2CDA, all have fewer side effects than other drugs currently in use. There is surprisingly little nausea; vomiting, generally no hair loss and they are very well tolerated. The biggest side effect is immunosuppression. Suppression of the immune system puts patients at risk for infections.

Amazingly, all of the various types of blood cells originate from a single type of cell, called the "pluripotential cell", which resides in the bone marrow. Some blood cells (like the pluripotential time) stay inside the bone marrow, while the more mature types (like red and white blood cells) are meant to circulate through the bloodstream, to go to wherever they are needed. Leukemia is usually a cancer of the white blood cells. It is divided into type general types, **Acute** and **Chronic.**

This distinction is based upon their untreated behavior-- with no treatment acute leukemias will kill within months, while chronic leukemia patients may live for many years. However, there is a flipside to this--**it is usually easier to cure acute leukemia than the chronic variety.**

Both acute and chronic leukemias are further sub classified as to the particular type of blood cell they arise from. White blood cells are larger than red blood cells and are easy to see under the microscope. Too few white blood cells ("leucopenia") lead to massive infections, with bacteria, viruses and fungi. Too few red blood cells lead to anemia, with pallor and weakness. Too few platelets lead to easy bruising and internal bleeding.

Acute leukemias, unlike the chronic variety, often have normal or decreased white blood cells. A hallmark of all leukemias is insufficient production of other normal blood cells, since the resources are being diverted to the leukemic cell population.

Another crucial distinction in leukemias besides "acute" and "chronic" is between the **Lymphocytic** and **Myelogenous** types. The Lymphocytic variety comes from lymphocytes, which is a common white blood cell active in identifying and marking germs to be killed.

In adults, about 1/3 of the total white blood cells are lymphocytes, and in young children up to 2/3 are lymphocytes. The Myelogenous variety comes from other blood cells besides lymphocytes, represents at least 7 different subtypes, and is often just called **"non-lymphocytic"** leukemia. These non-lymphocytic types may arise from the red blood cell line ("erythroleukemia") or from the platelet line ("megakaryocytic types").

Sometimes the types are found in combination that is the disease is composed of more than one type of leukemia. Also, as the disease gets more advanced, it may start showing other "clones" instead of the "pure type" that it started as.

The major divisions of acute and chronic, and lymphocytic and myelogenous, are combined into the following four labels into which all leukemias can be grouped:-

ALL (Acute Lymphocytic Leukemia)
AML (Acute Myelocytic Leukemia)
CLL (Chronic Lymphocytic Leukemia)
CML (Chronic Myelogenous Leukemia)

Sometimes a previous chronic leukemia will convert into the acute variety (called "Richter's syndrome") but since the clinical behavior and treatment of the acute and chronic types are different, they are considered as two separate topics. Like all cancers, leukemia starts from a **single** abnormal cell, and the type of cell will determine the type of leukemia. A change occurs in the genes of this cell that is in the information stored in the cells "DNA". Each body cell contains the information necessary to form a whole new body, but most of this is "masked" after the cell develops ("differentiates") into a particular adult cell type. The genes can be altered to command the cell to undergo uncontrolled division, and this is then cancer.

Ultimately, cancer is a disease of the DNA! Different recognized genetic abnormalities are found in the various subtypes of leukemia, this is an area of active research. Anyway, the abnormal cell makes billions of copies of itself, shunting resources away from normal cells division.

The "leukemic clone" takes over the bloodstream, choking off normal functioning and leading to the symptoms described below. If untreated, an acute leukemia is always fatal.

How Common is Acute Leukemia?

Combining childhood and adult cases, there are about 5,970 new cases of **ALL** (3,350 in males and 2,620 in females) & about 1,440 deaths from ALL (800 in males and 640 in females) in the U.S.A.

 Acute leukemia is the most common cancer of childhood. However, only 25% of the total cases occur in children. Overall, acute leukemia strikes 5 out of 100,000 people each year.

AML is 5 times more common than **ALL** but **ALL** represents 85% of cases in children. Thus, the average **ALL** patient is 4 years old while the average **AML** patient is 60 years old. If untreated, 95% of patients will die within one year of diagnosis.

The flipside of this is that most patients' disease free for over four years are likely cured (as contrasted with breast cancer which commonly re-emerges years after apparently successful therapy). Overall, the risk for leukemia has been increasing over 5 decades.

Regarding **AML** there are about 62,130 new cases of leukemia (all kinds) and 24,500 deaths from leukemia (all kinds).

New cases account for about 21,380 of **acute myeloid leukemia** (AML). Most will be in adults. There are 10,590 deaths from AML. Almost all will be in adults.

Acute myeloid leukemia is generally a disease of older people and is uncommon before the age of 45. The average age of a patient with **AML** is about 67 years.

AML is slightly more common among men than among women, but the average lifetime risk in both sexes is less than ½ of 1%.

What Causes or Increases the Risk for Acute Leukemia?

As for any cancer, the reason why one particular person gets acute leukemia and another does not remains **unknown.** However, some factors that markedly increase the chance for a person to get leukemia are well documented. "Primary" leukemia means it is the first blood cancer detected; "Secondary" leukemia arises detected; "Secondary" leukemia arises after treatment for some other cancer. Secondary leukemia is usually **AML** and develops an average of 5 years after treatment of another cancer. It is especially seen after treatment for Hodgkin's Disease, myeloma, lymphoma, breast or ovarian cancer. The more aggressive, the more likely later **AML** will occur.

Factors Increasing the Risk for Acute Leukemia:

1) Radiation Exposure is the best documented risk factor in adults. It causes genetic damage leading to various cancers. Fortunately, small amounts of radiation don't seem to cause leukemia, since exposure is inevitable from cosmic rays, radiation in our food (potassium-40) or emanating from metal deposits in the earth. Occasional X-rays **are not associated with leukemia**, but radiation therapy and atomic bomb exposure are.

2) Chemicals which increase cancer risk are called **"carcinogens"**. They also work through the mechanism of damage to genes. The best known chemicals associated with leukemia development are benzene, toluene, mustard gas and arsenic. **Drugs** related to these chemicals, such as the alkylating agents (from mustard gas) used to treat cancer, or chloramphenicol (phenol) as an antibiotic, are considered **"leukemogenic"** (causative of leukemias). Overall, chemotherapy is considered more strongly causative of Secondary leukemia than Radiation Therapy, and both together increase the risk greater than either one alone.

3) Heredity Conditions can include gene damage increasing risk for acute leukemias. Down's syndrome (3 chromosome #21's instead of the normal 2) increases risk, and siblings of leukemia patients have a 5 times higher risk. If one identical twin gets childhood leukemia, the chance that the other twin will get it is 25%. Bloom's syndrome patients have frequent chromosome breaks (the genes are packed along the much larger chromosomes).

Fanconi's syndrome and Ataxia-Telangiectasia are other uncommon conditions with chromosome damage which likewise have higher leukemia development.

4) Prior Chronic Leukemia: Over 80% of patients with Chronic Myelocytic Leukemia will develop Acute Myelocytic Leukemia in the terminal stage of their disease. These patients are predominantly adults, and this type of "leukemic transformation", called **"Blast Crises"**, is very hard to treat.

5) Prior Blood Diseases, particularly "myelodysplastic" syndromes, also called "Preleukemia" and "refractory anemias". These patients are usually over 50 years old, have abnormal blood smears, and a bone marrow which is always abnormal. These conditions may smolder for many years before becoming acute leukemia, about 30% of the time.

*** Viruses, Alcohol and Tobacco Use Haven't Been Linked to Acute Leukemia.

What are the Symptoms of Acute Leukemia?

Early Acute Leukemias will have no symptoms, as the "cancer cell burden" is insufficient to cause symptoms. As the "leukemic clone" multiplies and fills up the bone marrow, and then the circulating blood, the following symptoms may occur:

Symptoms and Signs of Acute Leukemia:

1) **Infection** is the most common presenting symptom (35%). This is because leukemic white blood cells don't work properly. Infections can be caused by bacteria, viruses, fungi, protozoans or parasites. Although everyone gets infections, leukemia patients get them more easily, and they tend to be harder to treat. Most patients who present with an infection have vague "flu-like" symptoms.

2) **Easy Bruising or Hemorrhage** (failure of the blood to clot). This is caused by a decrease in the number of circulating blood platelets, the fragments crucial to forming a clot. Low platelets ("thrombocytopenia") can show as internal bleeding, bruising or little purple bumps on the skin surface ("petechia").

3) **Fatigue and Paleness** caused by **anemia**, which is a decrease

in the number of red blood cells. About 80% of patients have some anemia, but it may be insufficient to cause symptoms.

4) Weight loss is seen in about 15% of patients. It takes lots of calories to keep the cancer cells growing.

5) Bone Pain is especially seen in **ALL** in children. As the leukemic clone fills up the bone marrow, it pushes on nerves causing pain.

6) Abdominal Swelling may be noticed by an increase in belt-size, and due to the leukemic cells filling up and stretching out the liver and spleen. This is more common with **ALL** than **AML**.

7) Glandular Swelling is caused by spread of the leukemia to lymph nodes. These are normally bean-sized kidney shaped glands which help filter blood to destroy germs. White blood cells are normally found in lymph nodes, but leukemic white cells fill them up and enlarge them. Enlargement can also result from infections. Boys may have testicular swelling from leukemia growth there.

8) Nervous System problems like vision impairment, mental deterioration or leukemic infiltration of the brain lining (meningitis) are rare but reported, especially in advanced stages of the disease.

It is important to note that all of the above symptoms are more commonly caused by other conditions besides leukemia, usually by persistent infections. The only way that leukemia can be absolutely diagnosed is via examination of blood and bone Marrow, as described below.

How is Acute Leukemia Diagnosed and Evaluated?

If a patient comes to medical attention with symptoms and signs of leukemia or some other serious blood disorder, the following are standardly done:

1) Complete Physical Examination looking for paleness, infection or bruising from lack of effective red cells, white cells and platelets respectively.

The liver and spleen are felt for enlargement, as well as the lymph gland clusters in the neck, armpit ("axilla") and groin. In males the testicles are examined for swelling, and a neurologic exam is done on all patients. Any new complaints such as fever, weight loss or night sweats are recorded.

2) Laboratory Tests include standard Complete Blood Count **("CBC")** that checks red blood cell count, white blood cells count, and platelets. Blood "smear" is made and the shapes of the blood cells are viewed under the microscope. This is the way that particular types of white blood cells are identified. The basic types are lymphocytes (30%), neutrophils (60%), Eosinophils (5%), Monocytes (3%) and Basophils (1%). Signs of infection include multi-segmented areas in the neutrophils, increased percentage of lymphocytes, or "toxic granulation" particles in these cells. Also, the actual number or white cells per cubic milliliter of blood is often above or below the normal value (4,000 - 10,000) with infections or leukemia.

It is important to remember that the blood smear from the circulating blood only gives an idea of what is going on in the bone marrow, which must be examined in to diagnose leukemia (see below). Also obtained is a Chemistry Panel **("SMA")** which tells blood sodium, potassium, bicarbonate, glucose, cholesterol, and liver and kidney function. Also, it tests for calcium, phosphorus and uric acid which may be abnormal. Tests of blood clotting ability are **PT**, **PTT** and bleeding time. A urinalysis **("UA")** tells about infection, blood, sugar or protein in the urine.

3) Radiology Tests include standard **Chest X-ray,** which shows pneumonia tumors in the chest. If the Chest X-ray is abnormal, a **CT scan** of the chest is commonly obtained. CT scans of the abdomen and pelvis, bone scans and brain scans are only obtained if there are symptoms in those areas.

4) Specialized Tests for Leukemia include **Bone Marrow Biopsy.** The biopsy means a special needle is stuck into the hip-bone, just above the buttock, and some marrow sucked out for examination. This is usually done on each side, since two samples are more accurate than one. It is done under local anesthesia and takes about 15 minutes. The bone marrow is placed in solution and a smear made upon a microscope slide.

By examining this slide, a pathologist can diagnose leukemia or other blood disorders, but not necessarily the specific subtype. We can see how many of the white blood cells are "blasts", that is new and presumably leukemic cells.

We can also see how many cells the bone marrow is producing, if it is overly full of cells, (which causes them to get deformed) or depleted of blood cells ("hypocellular"). Repeat tests of the bone marrow will be needed to gauge the effectiveness of therapy.

The first step is to distinguish between a lymphocytic or non-lymphocytic subtype, by looking at the cells to see if they are lymphocytes or not. The next step is to help rule-out the chance that an increased number of white blood cells are due to an infection -- that is a "leukemoid reaction". For this, a test called Lymphocyte (or Neutrophil) acid Phosphatase, **("LAP")** is done on the cells and the LAP score calculated. High LAP scores are more likely to mean infection. If "Auer Rods" are seen in the circulating cells, the disease will almost certainly be **AML.** Acute leukemia is likely if the "Philadelphia Chromosome" is seen, as it is in 10% of children and

30% of adults with **AML** or **ALL**.

There are particular staining techniques to identify the 7 subtypes of AML, the classifications of which are discussed below. A newer and more accurate way of classifying both **AML** and **ALL** is **"immunophenotyping"**. This means testing for surface cell markers produced by each specific type of leukemia. Immunophenotyping will tell at which stage of development the cell became leukemic, that is how "differentiated" it is.

This has important treatment implications, since more differentiated leukemias tend to need more treatment to eradicate them.

For lympho- cytic leukemias, immunophenotyping distinguishes between the **"B"** and **"T"** cell subtypes. This is important since the less common "T" cell subtype (20%) may require more aggressive treatment.

Spinal Tap is an important test to tell whether the fluid bathing the brain and spinal cord ("cerebral spinal fluid or **CSF** ") is invaded by leukemic cells. If so, then aggressive treatment will be mandatory to clear this area of disease. The spinal fluid, the brain linings it bathes ("meninges") and the testicles in males are considered **"sanctuary sites"** meaning that leukemic cells can hide there to escape regular treatment.

Thus, it must be ascertained if these areas are involved, with spinal tap and **testicular biopsy**, to see if they will need extra therapy to eradicate disease there. Since these areas are often the first site of relapse after treatment, continued monitoring of them after treatment is essential to detect any relapse early.

What are the Subtypes of Acute Leukemia?

In 1976, the French-American-British Cooperative Group **(FAB)** developed a system for classifying acute leukemias, which is in wide use

Copyright - 2017. Published by Cancer Group Institute. www.cancergroup.com 16

today. This classification is based upon the way the leukemic cells look under the microscope, and thus their presumed normal counterparts of origin.

For ALL L1 means the childhood form of ALL; lots of small lymphocytes.

L2 means the adult form of ALL; lymphocytes are larger.

L3 Burkitt's lymphoma-- rare-- most aggressive type. The most favorable type is L1; the least favorable is L3, with L2 intermediate. **ALL** can then be further sub classified by immunophenotyping, to see if the cells are **"B"** or **"T"** origin. Their surface proteins can be analyzed to determine how "mature" the cells are. For instance, **"B"** lymphocytes normally develop in a progression from **"early pre-B"** to **"pre-B"** to **"B"**; in general the less mature the lymphocyte the less "surface immunoglobulin" (protein) it produces, and the easier it is to treat successfully.

AML arises from any blood cell beside lymphocytes, so it's classification is even more complicated, and divided into 7 **"M"** categories by the **FAB** system, and followed by their relative proportions making up adult acute leukemia:

M1 "myeloblastic" cells, very immature can be confused with L2; 20%

M2 "myeloblastic" cells with maturation, larger cells, 30%

M3 "promyelocytic" cells are further developed than M1 or M2 10%

For AML M4 "myelomonocytic" more mature looking like monocytes 30%

M5 "monocytic"-- the cells look just like monocytes. 10%

M6 "erythrocytic" means it comes from red blood cell lineage <5%

M7 "megakaryoblastic" -- it comes from platelet making cells <5%
Sometimes the acute leukemias start off as one form and seem to develop into another. For instance, **M6**, "erythroleukemia", usually "progresses" to **M2** or **M4.** This occurs as the unstable DNA within the leukemic clone changes form. Also, the altered biochemical conditions fostered by one leukemic clone might encourage another different leukemia to arise, in the patient already predisposed to develop leukemias, and so more than one type may be seen in that patient.

What are the Factors Influencing Outcome in Leukemia?

Factors influencing predicted outcome and survival in disease are called "prognostic factors" and these have been identified for acute leukemia:
ALL worsening characteristics:

a) Types **L2** or**L3** as opposed to **L1**; production of mature surface proteins.
b) Being Male, or Adult (children ages 3 to 7 do best).
c) "T" cell leukemia as opposed to "B" cell.
d) High White Blood Cell count (over 25,000); severe anemia, low platelets.
e) Organ or Glandular swelling, mass in the center of chest ("mediastinum").
f) Involvement of the spinal fluid, brain linings, or eyes. ("CNS leukemia").
g) Presence of Philadelphia Chromosome, especially after treatment.

AML worsening characteristics:

a) Age older than 60 years, Down's syndrome, infant-age children.
b) Secondary **AML**, after treatment for **ALL** or another cancer.
c) **AML** arising out of a long standing "myelodysplastic" syndrome.

d) Presence of the Philadelphia Chromosome, especially after treatment.

What is the Survival From Acute Leukemia?

This will depend upon many factors, including the particular type of leukemia, the condition of the patient, and the therapy selected. According to textbooks, prior to discovery of chemotherapy everyone with acute leukemia died within 2 years. The following results are seen with *conventional therapy* still used today:

For **ALL,** the cure rate is currently 40% for adults and 60% for children. For **AML** the cure rate is currently 20%, overall.

No one can predict how long any individual patient will live; we are not "M. Deities". Recall that many patients live longer than expected, and lead high quality lives, with their cancer.

What is the Conventional Treatment for Acute Leukemia?

The most important thing in treating leukemia is the induction of a ***"complete remission"*** in the patient. A "complete remission" is defined as:
1) No sign of leukemic cells in the patients' blood or bone marrow, the bone marrow should have less than 5% "blasts" (young cells).

2) Normal white blood cell, red blood cell, and platelet counts.

3) No residual organ, testicle or glandular swelling.

4) Ability of patient to return to previous normal activities.

Unfortunately, **"complete remission"** does **not** mean getting rid of every last leukemia cell; it does mean there are too few to be detected with our current technology. In practice, the number of leukemia cells is probably reduced from a trillion to a billion with induction therapy. This is enough to resolve all symptoms.

After successful induction of remission, the next step is to **"consolidate"** the remission with **"intensification therapy"** given over several months. After this, the remission may be **"maintained"** with **"maintenance therapy"** spanning out over several years. Only after the patient has been kept in complete remission for several years can the total discontinuance of therapy be considered, although close follow up will be essential to at least 5 years.

Cancer doctors speak in terms of **"phases"** of therapy for leukemia-- **"induction, consolidation, intensification, maintenance"** to describe each stage of the treatment, and to be able to compare the results of various regimens.

The refinements in the treatment of leukemia have been by examining the results of side effects of each of these particular phases and trying to improve upon them. Improvement may actually mean that the therapy becomes *less* aggressive. For instance, radiation to the brain used to be used for most children with leukemia, but now is only used for those with high risk factors.

Treatment for acute leukemia always includes chemotherapy, and may additionally use radiation therapy, immune therapy, and bone marrow transplant. Preventative therapies ("prophylaxis") may be necessary for "sanctuary sites" (i.e. nervous system). Treatments used will depend upon the type of leukemia, how extensive it is the condition of the patient, and the available local facilities.

We will now consider the standard therapies for **ALL** and **AML:**

For ALL the standard "Remission Induction" phase is:

Vincristine and Prednisone will produce remission in 90% of children and 50% of adults. Each agent used alone is only half as effective. Adding ***L-asparaginase*** ups remission to 95%. in children and 80% in adults. ***Doxorubicin*** (adriamycin) can be added instead. The use of more than 3 drugs has not improved success rates. A bone-marrow biopsy after 7 days of treatment is useful to predict if the regimen is working. If it doesn't work by 6 weeks, there is no use continuing that particular therapy.

Side- Effects of ALL Remission Induction Drugs:

Vincristine derived from the periwinkle plant and given by injection. It can cause "peripheral neuropathy", meaning pain and numbness from nerve damage, as well as kidney damage and hearing loss. It lowers blood cell counts, which can lead to anemia and infection. The risk of these side effects depends upon the dose and what other drugs are being used. Many patients have minimal side effects. **Prednisone** is a cortisone derivative that can be taken as a pill.

This "steroid" drug reduces the white blood cell count, and over time will increase the risk for infection, thin bone, raise the chance of internal bleeding and cause a "Cushingoid" appearance (fat face and body, thin limbs, hair growth, 'buffalo hump' on back). It is usually very well tolerated over short courses (e.g. a few weeks), and the side effects become more prominent with higher doses over a longer time. **L-Asparaginase** is from the amino acid asparagine and is given into the veins ("I.V.").

It causes nerve damage and nausea. **Doxorubicin** (Adriamycin) is a brilliant red color "anthracycline" (from coal) and is always given I.V. It's main side-effect is heart damage (no more than 500 mg. per square meter of body area are given, and a heart test ("MUGA") is taken first. Also it can cause lung damage, and the skin to become redder than normal with radiation. It causes hair loss (usually temporary), and decreased blood counts.

For ALL the "Consolidation and Intensification" phase, and "Prophylaxis" is:

Cytarabine (ARA-C) with or without intermittent "pulses" of vincristine and prednisone. The idea here is to further reduce the presumed one billion or so leukemic cells remaining after remission induction.

CNS Prophylaxis is mandatory in children after complete remission and the methods of clearing the Central Nervous System of actual or presumed leukemia cells have been subject to much study. If no CNS prophylaxis is given to children, it will be the first site of relapse 50% of the time. While adolescents and adults usually get prophylaxis, it has not been shown to improve survival for them.

Previously radiation therapy used to be always used; it is now only used in high-risk patients and those with actual CNS leukemia. Instead, most patients get **"Intrathecal Chemotherapy"** -- directly into the spinal canal given with a spinal tap.

The drug most used is **Methotrexate.** In low risk patients, Methotrexate alone is sufficient therapy, reducing CNS relapse from 30% to just 5%. In those with high-risk disease, itis appropriate to add **"cranial"** radiation (10 treatments totaling 18.0 Gray) to reduce the CNS relapse risk from over 50% to 5%.

Treating the entire spinal column with radiation (in addition to the skull) used to be common, but this **"cranial-spinal"** irradiation is now almost always avoided since it is doesn't help survival, and causes growth deformity, nutrition problems, and bone marrow damage in children.

The only current use for cranial-spinal irradiation is to treat florid relapse in the CNS. In a patient receiving both Methotrexate and Radiation, it is *critical* to give the Radiation first, and then the Methotrexate, since this causes less brain damage than vice-versa.

***Side Effects of Consolidation and CNS Prophylaxis: Cytarabine (ARA-C)** can also be used in CNS prophylaxis for those not responsive to Methotrexate. It very powerfully lowers blood counts. It is given as an injection. It can cause liver and kidney damage. The side effects of the other drugs used for consolidation are above.

Cranial Irradiation: Is given to each side of the head, while using a block to protect the lens of the eye. It is also called "whole brain" irradiation. The treatment is given with a Linear Accelerator (Linac) with high-energy photons.

The therapy takes about 3 minutes per day for 10 days, Monday through Friday. The therapy itself if painless, small children may need short-acting anesthesia to hold still. Radiation causes the scalp hair to fall out (temporarily) and the patient to be tired during treatment.

Long term, children who receive radiation may develop a syndrome of acute fatigue and lethargy which slowly improves as the brain heals. They tend to have somewhat lower IQ scores and more propensities to behavioral problems, but it is hard to separate out the contributions of radiation, chemotherapy, and just the trauma of being diagnosed and treated for leukemia. Recent studies have shown no worse brain functioning in children who got both cranial radiation and methotrexate versus just methotrexate.

For ALL the "Maintenance" phase is: 6-Mercaptopurine (6-MP) used daily is added to oral methotrexate weekly, and sometimes with prednisone and the other drugs above. 6-MP is given as a pill, lowers blood counts and can cause some back up in the liver. The question of how long to continue maintenance is controversial, but in childhood ALL it's at least 30 months.

***Side-Effects of Maintenance Therapy:

6-MP and **Methotrexate** must be given in sufficient dose to lower blood counts ("**hematosuppression**") to be effective. This means the patient will be at risk for anemia and infections. Also, these drugs can cause mouth sores ("stomatitis"), diarrhea, and liver and kidney function (that must be closely monitored). Giving these drugs to children can cause growth problems and bone weakness ("**osteoporosis**").

As mentioned, children are often socially underdeveloped due to the stresses of the disease and its treatment.

For AML (except M3) the Remission Induction Drugs are: **Cytarabine**, **Idarubicin** or **Daunorubicin** are typical induction drugs.

It is mandatory to give these drugs until almost complete bone marrow shutdown, which occurs within 10 - 14 days after treatment begins. The regimen will need to be repeated if a complete remission is not gotten. About 75% of patients will have a complete remission within a month of starting treatment. However, this remission alone is temporary.

***Side effects of AML Remission Induction Drugs: **Cytarabine** and **Idarubicin** together are a very powerful combination.

The treatment lowers blood counts so drastically that the patient must be very carefully monitored for anemia, infection and internal bleeding.

Temporary baldness, nausea and vomiting, and mouth sores occur. The regimen can cause heart damage and even heart failure. A certain type of "port" (catheter) must be put into a major vein to give the drugs, and local tissue damage will occur if the drugs seep out of the port into the surrounding tissues.

The port itself is subject to infections and may "clot-off", necessitating putting through streptokinase or some other clot-dissolving agent. Not all patients can tolerate such aggressive induction; it is especially difficult on the elderly or very young.

The elderly may opt for lower doses of these drugs, or oral drugs like **hydroxyurea** which has a lower cure rate, but also less early deaths from therapy and better quality of life.

If the elderly do get the standard remission drugs in full doses, their remission rates are the same as for younger patients.

For AML type M3 (Promyelocytic) the Remission Induction Is: Trans-Retinoic Acid, a vitamin A derivative, given as pills twice per day for about 2 months. Nearly all patients get a complete remission, without problem of blood count lowering. However, after the remission standard intensive chemotherapy will still be needed (as described below) to help prevent relapse. The problem of inappropriate blood clotting is seen in over 80% of patients with the M3 type; this must be carefully monitored.

AML After-Remission Therapy:

It is essential to continue treating the patient with AML after a complete remission is obtained, since over 95% of patients would relapse without

Copyright - 2017. Published by Cancer Group Institute. www.cancergroup.com 25

more therapy. The appropriate treatment to maintain complete remission is dependent upon the condition, tolerance and wishes of the patient and what's available. The doses of drugs given may have to be reduced if they are causing excessive blood count lowering or otherwise sickening the patient.

In general, after remission therapy ("post-remission") is given after the patient's blood counts have recovered from the induction phase. The post-remission drugs are given for at least 4 cycles, but long-term "maintenance" chemotherapy has **not** been shown to improve survival, and definitely hampers quality of life. The drugs commonly used: *Cytarabine (ARA-C)* is given by vein alone or again in combination with a drug like **Daunorubicin**. While the duration for giving this treatment is controversial there is no question that patients who complete one or more "consolidation courses" (cycles) with these drugs have a longer survival than those who do not. These drugs severely depress blood counts, of both leukemic and normal cells, and some considerations of this are:

a) Replacement Therapy of critical blood components, that is transfusions, will be necessary if the hemoglobin drops below 8 or the platelets below 20,000. It gets harder to transfuse successfully as the patient develops antibodies to donor blood cells and platelets, and the immune system destroys them. If the white blood cell count falls to under 500 and the patient has a fever, they get l **"granulocyte transfusions"** and antibiotics.

b) Supportive Therapy includes giving proper nutrition and fluids to keep metabolism balanced, and drugs like Allopurinol which help excrete that excess uric acid released from killed blood cells, preventing it from building up and causing gout. A remarkable advance in support has been the development of **Growth Factors** which stimulate new blood cells to form, specifically **erythropoietin** to stimulate red blood cells and **neupogen** (GM-CSF) to stimulate white blood cell development. We are working on a growth factor to stimulate platelet growth, but don't have it yet. Giving growth factors can **reduce anemia and infections without transfusions.**

Results of Conventional Therapy for AML:

Without any treatment, the average survival for AML patients is just 3 months.

When giving chemotherapy, replacement and supportive therapy as described above, above, the average survival increases to about 18 months. This means some patients live much longer, and about 20% of patients are alive and disease free at 5 years. The most common causes of demise in patients are infections and hemorrhage resulting from the disease, its therapy, or both. The longest survivals from conventional treatment are from studies that use intensive consolidation chemotherapy after complete remission is achieved by induction.

Latest Effective Treatments for Acute Leukemia.

Bone Marrow Transplant is the most exciting practical development for both ALL and AML. We first describe the process and side effects, then the latest results. It is important to note that the success rates have been increasing, and the complication rates decreasing, as more Bone Marrow Transplants are done. While the procedures used to be limited to only the most advanced University Hospitals, there is now a push for some to be done at smaller Community Hospitals given increased safety and success with experience and new drugs.

The rationale for Bone Marrow Transplant is that it allows much higher doses of chemotherapy to be given than otherwise possible, wiping out not only the cancer cells but also the patient's entire ability to manufacture new blood cells. If the blood-forming cells were not replaced, this would be lethal.

Basically, Bone Marrow transplant is merely a method of replacing the blood forming cells after intensive chemotherapy. There are two distinct types of Bone Marrow Transplant, the first being using the patient's own blood forming cells which have been **"harvested"** and stored **("autologous transplant")** and the second is using "donor" blood-forming cells from another person **("allogeneic transplant")**.

When using donor blood forming cells, the donor is usually a very close relative since the cells must be closely matched to those of the patient, for the transplant to a success. To match marrow a sample must be taken by needle, usually from a hip bone, and the sample is **"HLA matched"** see how similar it is to the patients.

Only identical twins would have identical marrow, but the closer of a match that can be obtained, the less chance for rejection in the patient. Using donor marrow is fraught with more difficulties than using the patient's own stored marrow, so "autologous" transplants are generally preferred, provided the patient's stored marrow can be "purged" of the leukemic clone.

It makes no sense to give the patient back his own leukemia cells and re-initiate the disease! For both autologous and allogeneic transplants, there are **two** basic ways that the blood-forming cells can be collected.

The first and older technique is to "harvest" bone marrow from the iliac wing bones, which are found in the hip area. The patient or matched donor is taken to the operating room and commonly put under general anesthesia.

About 50 punctures are made with a special bone-boring needle into the bone above each buttock, and the marrow from this area sucked out ("aspirated").

There is no significant danger (besides anesthesia risk) to the donor, this marrow is expendable, but some scarring is common in the harvest area. The marrow is stored in glass jars. If it comes from the patient, then it may be cleaned ("purged") of leukemia cells; this process is unnecessary if it comes from a healthy donor.

New techniques have improved the success of purging, but it still remains a risk to give the patient back there their disease in the transplant. **The second and newer method** is less invasive and does not take actual marrow, but instead **"stem cells"** circulating in the bloodstream. These "stem cells" can form new marrow, all crucial blood cells, and they "reconstitute" the blood.

For stem-cell collection, the procedure is *not* called a "Bone-Marrow" transplant but instead a "Peripheral Stem Cell Transplant". Since currently this procedure is used with patient's own stem cells, the full name is "**Autologous Peripheral Stem Cell Transplant".**

For this, the patient comes in several times and has a needle ("catheter") inserted into an arm vein. Blood is drawn out and processed through a special machine which collects stem cells, and then returns the residual blood back to the patient.

The cells removed are centrifuged to remove the circulating stem cells, which are packaged and stored. The process of separating specific white blood cells is called "leukophoresis" and ideally will remove the cancerous clone, while preserving the healthy stem cells to re-infuse. The next step for any Bone Marrow Transplant is for the patient's own marrow to be destroyed by **chemotherapy** ("cytotoxic marrow ablation"). This is to annihilate the leukemic clone, and as a consequence destroys every other blood-forming cell at the same time.

Sometimes, part of the "preparative regimen" for Bone Marrow Transplant is the addition of **"whole body radiation"**. For this, the patient is sent down to the Radiation Oncology Department for initial measurements of body thickness, and to make appropriate physics calculations. During the Marrow Ablation phase (and while receiving the chemotherapy) about 6 whole body radiation treatments are given over 3 days (so two treatments per day about 6 hours apart).

The patient, on a cart, is usually placed against a wall in the treatment room and the Linear Accelerator is turned on for about 10 minutes per treatment. They are commonly treated from each side, with their arms at their sides to help lower the dose to the lungs.

A plexiglass "scatter screen" is placed between the patient and the machine, which helps boost up the dose to the skin. This is because leukemic cells can hide in the lower skin layers. The actual radiation treatment is painless, and the patient is then returned to their room.

The **side-effects** of the "preparative regimen" for Bone Marrow Transplant are due to a killing of all the rapidly dividing cells in the body. The side-effects will depend on whether just chemotherapy is used, or whether whole-body radiation is added also.

The chemotherapy side-effects are the same as noted above for when these drugs are used a primary treatment, but for marrow ablation higher doses are given. The dose is, in fact, "super-lethal", since the patient will die if the bone marrow is not replaced. The first cells to disappear from the bloodstream are those with the shortest normal life-- white cells often only live 10 hours! Next, the platelets, with an average life of 10 days, will disappear, and finally the red blood cells with an average life of 120 days.

Thus, if not replaced, we would expect to see, in order, infection, hemorrhage, and then anemia develop from the marrow ablative therapy. In practice, the patient will not live long enough to develop anemia, first dying from infection and hemorrhage. It takes a while for the re-infused bone marrow or stem cells to "take", and start producing new blood cells. This is a critical time for supportive transfusions and preventing infections.

The side effects of **whole body radiation** are divided into **"acute"** and **"late"** categories. **Acute** reactions, seen during the treatment period, include nausea, vomiting, and swelling of the salivary glands (looks like mumps), sore throat, hair loss and fatigue. Some skin redness may develop. These acute reactions will resolve with time.

Late reactions take weeks to years to manifest and include sterility, a thickening of the skin, cataract formation of the eyes, and possible heart, lung and liver damage. The most worrisome possible complications are "radiation pneumonitis" from overdose to the lungs, and "veno-occlusive" disease of the liver. These may range from mild to fatal.

The treatment is broken up into about 6 "fractions" to help reduce the risk of these late reactions, which used to be much more common when the whole treatment was given at one sitting. It is sometimes hard to thresh out which side effects came from the chemotherapy and which from radiation. Generally, however, the preparative regimen is well tolerated, and the patient can be supported with anti-nauseates and other medicines for comfort.

Once the "preparative" regimen has been completed, the stored blood-forming cells are infused into an ordinary vein. They circulate through the bloodstream and find their way into the center of the bones, sticking onto the bone "spicules" there.

They (hopefully)**"engraft"**, meaning take and start forming new blood cells. If they don't, the patient will die of "aplastic anemia" unless given constant transfusions. Happily, the cells do usually take, although new blood cell formation may at first be a very slow process.

The patient is given antibiotics to prevent infection, and daily blood counts are taken to check for engraftment. If the transplant is from another person ("allogeneic") who is not an identical twin, then anti-rejection drugs like Cyclosporine and Thymosin will be given to help prevent rejection.

An unusual situation may arise when people are given foreign bone marrow. Instead of the body rejecting the transplant, as is seen with kidney or liver transplants, *the transplanted bone marrow rejects the body it is put into!* This is called **"Graft** versus **Host Disease**, or **"GVH"** for short. GVH manifests as skin rashes, fatigue and organ swelling, and low blood counts.

Sometimes a liver or skin biopsy is necessary to make the diagnosis. It is treated by increasing the amount of anti-rejection drugs the patient receives. Ironically, some GVH actually helps ensure that the transplant is a success, by killing off any remaining leukemic cells in the patient's body!

Thus, doctors may not wish to suppress GVH totally, although it can be fatal if it is uncontrolled. Normally, patients are ready to go home after several weeks in the hospital, and can return to regular activities. If the patient relapses after bone-marrow transplant, it can be tried again, but the whole body radiation is only given once in the life of each patient, either on the first transplant or afterward.

In conclusion, new technology like growth factors, retinoin, bone-marrow transplant and anti-rejection drugs are giving more hope than ever to patients with acute leukemia. It is crucial to get an opinion from doctors at a University Academic Medical Center, familiar with open protocols you may wish to participate in.

Acute Leukemia is an aggressive disease, which requires aggressive therapy. It is advisable to take a multi-faceted approach, and not just rely upon the conventional treatment. This means not only listening to an oncologist you trust for the primary treatment, but also taking an active role in the therapy.

A reasonable alternative therapy, which is not overtly toxic or overly expensive, should be sought as well as programs of nutrition and exercise. "Mind over Cancer" thoughts can be helpful, along with keeping a positive attitude, even in the face of setbacks.

Studies have shown than patients with positive attitudes and a strong will to live do better than those who have a depressed and complacent attitude. Living each day fully, and using all the tools available to fight the disease, will enhance your quality of life, and give you the peace-of-mind knowing that you have done everything possible to help ensure a happy outcome.

You Don't Have to Settle for Conventional "Strategies of Containment" About the best that spokespersons for the conventional cancer establishment can say in summarizing more than 25 years of cancer research is: "we're making headway."

This publication summarizes the physicians and alternative health experts that have an altogether different view. You don't have to settle for strategies of containment while you wait for scientists to discover that single magical cure for cancer. The treatments summarized in this publication offer clinical proof-drawn from patient case records of successful multi modal alternative approaches to cancer. None of the physician's treatments in this packet will ever speak in terms of a "single cure" for cancer. Medically, this is a sophomoric notion, not founded in physiological realities.

This publication gives an overview of multiple treatments and substances working together -synergistically - to effect major changes in the cancer process, from containment to remission to a life that is cancer free.

"Synergy" in alternative medicine treatments means many substances work cooperatively in such a way as to enhance the overall effect, making it stronger than single substances could ever produce alone. More important, even though there are dismaying cancer statistics, you or anyone you know does not have to become a statistic.

Cancer reversal is quite possible, but it requires some effort, some personal commitment and trust on the part of the others involved, and a comprehensive knowledge by the physician or alternative health practitioner of the modalities available and their effectiveness as proven in clinical practice.

Mortality from certain cancers may seem statistically likely, but that is an illusion compounded by fear and ignorance. It's not only patients who fear cancer outcomes; probably most oncologists are equally in fear of this disease and shield themselves against the disturbing scenarios, statistics, and probabilities they know too well.

The physician's treatments researched in this publication offer patients the statistics of optimism. Men and women can and do survive cancer, and go on to live long, productive, healthy lives, hopefully, cancer free. This publication will provide an overview of select alternative treatments. First we will examine dietary support, then botanicals and supplements that fight cancer, followed by treatments for specifically neutralizing cancer and tumors.

There are many more additions to what we present and we hope that you will take action to win the battle over cancer by contacting a health professional to help you begin an alternative program, such as the physicians and alternative centers listed at the end.

Here is an example of the cancer process and its reversal by the person most affected - a man with cancer. Leukemias, which form in the blood and bone marrow are not solid tumors but are characterized by an overproduction of abnormal white blood cells. They travel through the bloodstream creating problems in the spleen and other tissues. Often, the root cause of the blood abnormality must be found.

Theodore, aged 50 came to Dr. Jesse Stoff, mentioned several times in this publication and listed at the bottom, with a diagnosis of chronic lymphocytic leukemia. His doctors urged bone marrow transplant and high dose chemotherapy, but he wanted none of that. Dr. Stoff's blood test showed that his bone marrow was being attacked by cytomegalovirus, which is a **herpes virus** often active in people with compromised immune systems. It triggered malignant changes in Theodore's bone marrow, which produced the leukemia. Dr. Stoff focused his therapy on treating the virus.

He gave a series of injectable remedies, including iscucin (made from Viscum album, or mistletoe, mentioned later) to stimulate the immunity.

He was then given once a day intravenous infusions of nutrients including vitamins C, B12, B6, calcium chloride magnesium, B complex, adrenal cortex extract and licorice extract. He also prescribed him many oral supplements of immune boosters including Super Colloidal Silver, folic acid and acidolphilus.

Next he gave him high nitrogen amino acids to help the natural killer cells neutralize the cancer, green tea extract and gamma linolenic acid.

This approach paid off for Theordore. His lymphocyte count dropped from 60,000 to 11,000 but it did take a whole year to reduce his white blood cell count to 20,000, at which point his nutritionals were changed by Dr. Stoff. Six months after his therapy change his virus was gone and he was in remission. He still takes supplements and receives the Iscucin injections for 6 weeks twice a year.

Therapies and Vaccines to Combat Leukemia Immuno-Augmentative Therapy:-

A biologist and cancer researcher named Lawrence Burton, Ph.D., has developed an alternative cancer therapy called **IAT.** He identified and isolated blood protein components that he suspected were associated with the development of cancer.

One of these, called C3 complement, activates two tumor antibodies, one is a deblocking protein factor. According to his theory, when the four blood components are balanced, the body can subdue cancer cells as part of its normal activity, if any of them are not balanced, the body's cancer defenses drop.

Dr Burton, discovered that by injecting certain amounts of these components into the patients, remissions of many types of cancer would occur, including some labeled as terminal. It is not a cure for cancer, however, it is more like a controller of cancer, much like insulin is for diabetes. IAT has achieved tumor reduction and even complete remission according to Dr. Burton in 40 to 60% of the patients who received it.

Since IAT is builds on the body's anticancer immune function, it is virtually nontoxic. The survival rate of Dr. Burton's patients were found to be approximately double the maximum survival rate of conventionally treated patients who had metatstatic cancers, from a study he completed of 79 patients with advanced cancers.

For more information on Immuno Augmentative Therapy, contact the IAT Center, PO Box F-42689, Freeport, Grand Bahama, Telephone: 242-352-4755.

TVZ-7 Lymphocyte Treatment:-

TVZ-7 is an example of a specific immunotherapy. This technique consists of culturing and harvesting B lymphocytes, a form of white blood cells that produce antibodies which neutralize foreign and dangerous matter in the blood. The extracted material, consisting of immune molecules which include interferons, interleukins and tumor necrosis factor are called TVZ-7, and is administered intravenously in 44-50 treatments during two weeks.

It is utilized mainly in other countries and by Canadian physicians, who see remarkable results with cancers of the blood, pancreas, skin, reproductive organs, colon, liver brain and gallbladder.

For more information on TVZ-7, contact Integrated Biologics Ltd., Biotechnology Research and Development. 130 Commerce Way, Woburn, MA 01801, Telephone 617-938-9088 or Dr. Ravi Devgan of Ontario,

Canada Telephone 416-487-0882.

Autogenous Bacterial Vaccine.

This is based on a form-changing microbe identified by Virginia Livingston, M.D. called *P.cryptocides*, which is found in high concentrations in cancer patients. It is described by her as a hidden killer and a lethal bloodstream infection that shows no direct signs of its existence. She developed a way to administer a vaccine made from the patient's own bacteria to fight this cancer microbe.

It is normally present in everyone, but is kept at bay by the immune system. When immunity is suppressed by poor diet, stress, chemical toxins, and many other factors, what normally is a dormant microbe can multiply and promote the growth of tumors. This microbe was identified in very high concentrations in cancer patients.

This vaccine is made by the bacteria in the person's body and fights the same bacteria, therefore the vaccine precisely matches each individual. They also contain vitamins and minerals to strengthen the immune system. It is given every 3 to 5 days, depending on the patient.

Other researchers report positive results with the Livingston vaccines, with no adverse reaction except for an occasional rash. For more information on this, contact The Livingston Foundation Medical Center 3232 Duke Street, San Diego, CA 92110, Telephone 619-224-3515.

Immuno-Placental Therapy (IPT)

This therapy was pioneered by Russian immunologist Valentine I. Govallo, M.D. He is the director of the Moscow Medical Institute's Laboratory of Clinical Immunology. The premise is that cancer had a specific immunologic character that allows it to evade attack by the human immune system.

Dr. Govallo discovered that this special factor is found in the human placenta, and he developed a vaccine from placental blood after live human birth to give the cancer patients immune system the ability to overpower the cancer and it's **"cloaking device."**

Other vaccines are very specific to certain types of cancer. Sometimes the body's same ability to cause tumor cells to die may also turn off the body's immune response to foreign tissues. In these cases tumor cells can gain advantage over the anti-cancer responses of the body.

Dr. Govallo's vaccine takes the human placenta factors that appear to suppress the defense mechanism of malignant cells, effectively allowing the tumor to be attacked and killed off. His approach is called IPT, but is widely known asVG-1000. It has been used effectively in the treatment of advanced cancers, with survival rates noted from his studies of over 20 years. The only side-effect seems to be an occasional fever and fatigue for 1-2 days. It is not indicated for the treatment of liver cancer, but is highly effective for most forms of early and advanced cancers.

Contact People Against Cancer, Box 10, Otho, IA 50569, Telephone 515-972-4444 for more information.

Botanical Cancer Medicines for Leukemia.

Astragalus
This botanical medicine has captured the interest of many conventional doctors because of its ability to reduce the toxic effects of conventional cancer treatment. It appears to protect the liver against the harmful toxic effects of chemotherapy and may be very effective in treating terminally ill liver cancer patients. A study in Peking Cancer Institute observed a much higher survival rate among advanced liver cancer patients when they were treated with both radiation and astragalus compared to those treated with radiation alone.

Echinacea

This is a well-known immune-enhancing herb. It was found to increase NK (natural killer) cell activity by 90% in patients with inoperable, far-advanced liver cancer when echinacea was combined with a thymus-stimulating agent (thymostimulun).

Also a natural chemical in Echinacea, arabinogalactin, stimulates the tumor-killing activity of macrophages. One of Echinacea's primary roles is to provide protection against infection, a common and sometimes deadly complication in advanced-stage cancers.

Cesium
A non-radioactive form of cesium, a rare alkali metal widely distributed in the Earth's crust and listed in the periodic table of elements, it has been used with success as an alternative cancer therapy. It has been suggested that cesium alkalanizes the body fluids and this, in turn, pushes the normally acidic (low) pH of the cancer cell toward a weakly alkaline (high) pH, promoting the cancer's demise. Thus cesium emerged as a high pH-inducing therapy.

A study reported that cesium chloride, when combined with chelation therapy (a method of binding an organic substance known as a chelating agent to a metallic ion with a positive electric charge [heavy metal] and removing it from the body) and nutritional supplements, led to significant improvement in about half of all "terminal" cancers of the pancreas, colon, gallbladder, liver, breast, prostate, and others most of which had not responded to conventional therapy.

Shark Cartilage.

Another protocol of treatment for cancer is shark cartilage, mentioned later in this publication. In 1994, the FDA granted Dr. Charles Simone an Investigational New Drug approval for his treatment of advanced cancers using this substance. Is contains angiogenesis inhibitors, which cut off the blood supply to tumor growth, thereby inhibiting new tumors.

During the clinical trial, he saw 100 patients with various advanced cancers. Some chose only the intensive shark cartilage program and his cancer-fighting plan, and some chose his plan in addition to chemotherapy. Complete remissions occurred in 3 patients. All the patients in the first group and half of the second experienced better energy levels, less pain, enhanced appetite, and more positive moods. Shark cartilage supplements can be purchased through the mail from any vitamin and supplement store that does mail orders.

Urea

A natural by-product of protein digestion and a natural diuretic, this substance has strong anticancer properties. When given orally, urea reaches high enough concentrations in the liver to inhibit cancer growth. Dr. Evangelos Danopoulos, from Athens, Greece found in the 1970's, that oral administration of urea was effective against liver cancer. In a study of 18 patients who were given urea orally 4-6 times per day, the patients survived an average or 26.5 months, 5 times longer than expected. A separate study with 11 patients with primary liver cancer and 17 with metastatic liver cancer yielded the same excellent results.

Green Concentrates.

Known as "green drinks" or the "super-vitamin," green concentrates can include chlorella, wheat and barley grass, spirulina, blue-green algae, and alfalfa. One called ProGreens is a dry green powder containing 33 nutritional substances, taken with water or juice, 1-2 times a day. The benefits, according to ProGreens, include immune support, antioxidant protection, gastrointestinal fortification, energy boosting, and overall nutrient supplementation, all extremely important to fighting cancer and its harmful effects. ProGreens can be contacted in San Leandro, CA at 510-639-4572. There is also Green Magic from New Spirit Naturals in San Dimas, CA 800-922-2766.

Other Botanicals worth looking into for their strong cancer fighting ability are Essiac, Garlic, Grape Seed Extract, Green Tea, Haelan 851, a liquid soybean concentrate, HANSI, a series of homeopathically prepared herbs, and Pau D' Arco, a herbal extract from the bark of South American *Tahebuia* trees, and others mentioned later in this publication.

Injectable Substances Which Help Combat Leukemia.

Ukrain.

This substance is derived from a combination of a common weed called clendine (chelidonium majus) and thiophosphoric acid, one of the original chemotherapeutic agents. This combination appears to neutralize the toxic effect of the alkaloids contained the plant. By this method, Ukrain has been rendered almost completely nontoxic, and fortified the body's tissues and anticancer defenses. It is a potent anticancer agent and also very safe. Like chemotherapy, it kills cancer cells very well, but unlike chemotherapy, it spares normal, healthy tissue. Ukrain can be purchased from Nowicky Pharma Margaretenstrasse 7 A-1040Vienna, Austria.

Telephone # 011 43 1 586 1224 Fax 011 43 1 586 8994 Email add, norwicky@Ukrin.com Mr. Hodish speaks understandable english. Ukrain should not be used with the drug Dexamethason (Dacradron) because it contains cortisone, which neutralizes the Ukrain.

Amygdalin/Laetrile.
This substance is highly concentrated in the pits of apricots, peaches, cherries, and berries. It is one of a group called nitrilosides, and has been found to have strong cancer-fighting potential, particularly with regard to secondary cancers, including a 60% reduction in lung metastases. It appears to neutralize the oxidative cancer-promoting compounds such as free radicals, which is just one more key component for keeping cancer from growing or spreading, and is considered entirely safe to use.

Tissue Extracts.

When taken orally or by injection, glandular and organ tissue extracts migrate directly to the gland or organ from which they are derived to provide support to that particular area and to help it fulfill its body-regulating and balancing functions.

Thymus extracts in particular, containing the thymus hormone called thymosin, have demonstrated effectiveness in treating cancers in both human and animal studies. In an animal study of lung cancer, a combination of thymosin and interferon (a natural immune system secretion) caused a "dramatic and rapid disappearance of tumor burden.

The animals treated with thymosin had stronger natural killer cell activity and lived significantly longer than those receiving standard chemotherapy. In trials involving people with lung cancer, patients receiving thymosin had significantly prolonged survival times relative to the other treatment groups.

To receive information on any of these and other substances, contact one of the alternative physicians or centers listed at the bottom of this publication.

Enzymes for Digestive Support.

Enzymes are fundamental to all living processes in the body, necessary for every chemical reaction and the normal activity of our organs, tissues, fluids, and cells. There are hundreds of thousands of these Nature's "workers." Enymes are specialized living proteins that enable your body to digest and assimilate food. There are special enzymes for digesting proteins, carbohydrates, fats, and plant fibers. Protease digests protein, amylase digests carbohydrates, lipase digests fats, cellulase for fiber and disaccharidase for sugars (Disaccharidases are enzymes that break down complex sugars (like lactose) into simple sugars (like glucose) so that the intestine can absorb the nutrients)..

When one has cancer, there is a usually a lack of enzymes and/or enzyme dysfunction. This creates an inability for the body to metabolize protein, which may promote cancer. This inability can be linked to improper amounts of proteolytic (protein-digesting) enzymes such as pepsin from the stomach and proteases from the pancreas which, along with hydrochloric acid **(HCI)** in the stomach, which are the body's first defense against cancer. Enzyme therapy can is an important step in restoring health and well-being by helping to remedy digestive dysfunction. Both plant-derived enzymes and animal-derived pancreatic enzymes are used in enzyme therapy.

One should seek to supplement with a whole food supplement that provides both nutrition and enzymes.

An overview of cancer markers.

A Cancer "Marker" generally refers to any of a variety of standard laboratory blood tests used to measure the level of a protein material or other chemical produced by cancer cells. These numbers become elevated in the presence of a cancer or tumors. X-rays and CT scans are cancer markers also, because they can determine the location of cancer in the body, but the term usually indicates a blood test.

Dr. Jesse Stoff, who is noted along with several other alternative physicians at the end of this publication, has observed that cancer markers do not always provide the best indication of the specific character or relative aggressiveness of a cancer. With breast cancer, for example, there are 4 different cancer markers, but it is rare to find a breast cancer that produces more than 2 or 3 of them. "You can have a huge tumor sitting there and any one of these markers can be well within normal range," Dr. Stoff says.

There is also a less than adequate correlation between cancer markers and the tumor mass. "You can have people with advanced metastatic disease and only moderately elevated levels of cancer markers, and vice versa," Dr. Stoff says. However, consistent correlations between tumor mass and cancer markers can serve as a rough approximation by how well the battle is going for any one individual, he adds.

When the treatment activates the immune system to respond to the tumor cells, the cancer markers will typically start showing a sudden rise or spike. This is because large amounts of proteins (tumor antigens, or cancer markers) are released as the cancer cells begin to die. "The cancer markers will go through the ceiling at this point," Dr. Stoff says. 'One needs to be prepared for this from a psychological point of view." If blood tests are done, cancer patients should realize that the rise will be transient and that it will drop precipitously, usually within 1 to 6 weeks.

During this period, the immune system's scavenging cells, the macrophages, will sweep up the cancer cells' debris. "The take-home lesson is that if you look at cancer markers only, you may get an inaccurate picture of how the cancer is behaving at that time," says Dr. Stoff. "The test should be repeated later on to ensure that the original reading is truly a spike, not an absolute, prolonged rise in the cancer markers."

Third, Dr. Stoff creates a list of all treatment options that may apply or "make biological sense" for this particular cancer. For Dr. Stoff, this may include alternative and conventional treatments as well as combinations of both that might maximize the clinical outcome while minimizing toxic side effects. Many patients treated by alternative physicians have already received extensive conventional treatment and are typically in need of intensive detoxification and immune-enhancing measures.

It is at the point where the cancer patient wants to combine effective strategies for an individual approach to their particular cancer that they should consult an alternative physician clinic, such as the one listed at the bottom of this publication, or a qualified holistic health nutritionist. These professionals will use the cancer markers to individually treat and change the treatments appropriately to maximize cancer elimination results.

Dietary Support for Cancer Patients.

A primarily vegetarian diet is the optimal nutritional strategy for supporting recovery from cancer, determined by objective laboratory tests (blood tests for nutrients, enzymes, hormones, and immune parameters) and subjective measures, such as a person's food tastes and willingness to try a new diet. Some hormone free chicken and high quality fresh fish can be eaten with (if possible to find) organic vegetables and high quality whole grains, legumes, fruits and nuts. If possible, begin to buy these foods at a local health food market if you are not already doing so.

The digestive capacities of the individual also must be considered, for they play a fundamental role in determining the body's usage of nutrients. Many cancer patients have a weakened digestive system, due to the cancer itself or, more often, the toxic effects of previous treatment by radiation or chemotherapy. Cooking foods helps because heating the food breaks down the cellulose, making nutrients more available for digestion.

"We usually begin with foods that are basically predigested, such as cooked grains and cooked vegetables, since the cancer patient's enzyme production in the small intestine is typically poor," Dr. Stoff says. "To consume raw vegetables or vegetable juices will cause additional stress because the patient won't digest it or absorb it. To support the digestive system I often recommend an enzyme formula called **Absorbaid**."

Vegetables can be cooked by quick steaming, being careful not to overcook, and only whole grains should be cooked and eaten. If one feels they can consume a moderate amount of raw vegetables and especially raw juices, it can make an immediate difference, flooding the body with essential cancer fighting nutrients.

Nutritionals to Add For a Cancer Fighting Diet.

This is a general overview of nutritionals, and there are many more. They idea is to begin to supplement with these and others prescribed by a qualified nutritionist so that the body can get a much needed boost in fighting cancer. One reason a cancer patient may feel so ill during conventional treatments is that the accumulation of the cancer cells' cellular debris is built up in the body in high levels. If the body does not eliminate these toxins, a patient can feel sick, nauseous, achy, have headaches, and flu-like symptoms. The only way to clear this up is through adequate nutrition and proper elimination. One must make sure to intake all the nutrients below, drink plenty of water, and look into certain types of toxicity-reducing enemas given by a qualified alternative practitioner.

Acidophilus.

A generic term for the Lactobacilli, "friendly bacteria" naturally inhabits the healthy intestine. It is very important to cancer therapy for these reasons: It exerts direct activity against cancers, it prevents cancer by detoxifying and preventing the formation of carcinogenic chemicals, reduces cholesterol which indirectly aids cancer resistance, helps produce important B vitamins, and curbs or destroys potentially pathogenic bacteria and hostile yeasts such as Candida albicans, resulting in freeing the immune system to fight cancer cells, and of great importance, through producing lactic acid, preserve and enhance the digestibility of foods which are fermented with them, such as soy products, sauerkraut, pickles and more.

L. acidophilus can significantly lower the cancer-triggering activity of compounds in the feces of persons who eat meat.

Amino Acids.

These create protein, and are also important to cancer therapy. Humans make 12 of these, but must ingest 8 of the essential ones. Some, our body makes under stress situations, but cannot make enough and it will benefit the body greatly to supplement with one such as glutamine. A test called a fasting plasma sample determines amino acid deficiencies, and if any our lacking, they can be added.

Particular amino acids beneficial in cancer treatment are L-arginine, which enhances NK cells, cytoxic T cells and others, Methionine, which should be taken with choline, Cysteine, which assists in detoxification and reduces side effects of chemotherapy and radiation.

Beta Carotene.

This is converted to vitamin A when the body needs it. Is an antioxidant and immune-enhancing supplement that has properties not found in vitamin A.

Calcium.

Taken with magnesium is very important, particularly for bone metastasis or bone cancers. There is a study that found that calcium deficiency was associated with a higher risk of colorectal cancer. Humans rarely get enough calcium into their diet, and supplementing with it should be for everyone.

Chromium.

Taken as either Chromium (III) picolinate or chromium polynicotinate, this may help people regain normal thyroid function, which can then bolster thyroid function. It also helps regulate blood sugar levels and this can substantially improve immune function and cancer resistance. Refined foods such as white sugar and flour are nutritionally defunct of chromium, unlike whole grains, and these substances can also deplete the body of chromium.

Coenzyme Q10 (COQ10).

Also known as ubiquinone, it is essential for generating energy in living things that use oxygen. The body produces some coQ10, but less with aging, and eating foods that contain it is very important, such as fish, especially sardines, soybean and grapeseed oils, sesame seeds, pistachios, walnuts, and spinach.

When combines with vitamin E, selenium, and beta-carotene, coQ10 can significantly reduce free-radical damage in the liver, kidney and heart tissues. Some recent findings show that supplementation with coQ10 can cause complete regression of tumors in advanced breast cancer.

Copper.

A trace element that is essential to proper functioning of a many immune cell types which fight and defend against cancer. It is vital to healing processes, excretion of toxins, forming red blood cells, and maintaining connective tissues. It is important to resist infections and also affects inflammation.

Eicosapentenoic Acid (EPA Fish Oils)- Essential Fatty Acids These are required for proper metabolism. They include linoleic and alpha linolenic acid and are found in flaxseed oil, certain seeds, nuts and vegetables. They are important in reducing heart disease and prevention and treatment of various cancers. It is very important to assist they body to fight cancer with the supplement flaxseed oil, which exerts a strong anticancer effect, and animal studies show 50% reductions in tumor size after 1-2 months of supplementation.

Green Concentrates.

Known as "green drinks" or the "super-vitamin," green concentrates can include chlorella, wheat and barley grass, spirulina, blue-green algae, and alfalfa. One called ProGreens is a dry green powder containing 33 nutritional substances, taken with water or juice, 1-2 times a day. The benefits, according to ProGreens, include immune support, antioxidant protection, gastrointestinal fortification, energy boosting, and overall nutrient supplementation, all extremely important to fighting cancer and its harmful effects. ProGreens can be contacted in San Leandro, CA at 510-639-4572. There is also Green Magic from New Spirit Naturals in San Dimas, CA 800-922-2766.

Botanicals That Fortify The Immune System.

There are a wide range of botanicals, and we will evaluate two that are noted to be indispensable to effective cancer treatment. Iscador (known as European mistletoe or Viscum album) and Larix (or Arabinogalactan). These botanicals work in a complementary fashion to support the body's anticancer defenses.

Iscador- From the holistic point of view, Iscador's unique therapeutic value, its specific effect on tumors, lies in its ability to counteract the disorderly spread of the carcinoma. According to Hans Richard Heiligtag, M.D., this action results from mistletoe's "strict formative force which expresses itself in its regular rhythmical growth, and on the other hand in its special relation to light and warmth, which enables it to blossom in wintertime. These three factors enable mistletoe to be a cancer remedy.

In other words, the strong force counteracts the revolt of the forces which characterize the malignant cell. At the same time, the ability to counteract the cold of wintertime carries over into mistletoe's ability to counteract the "coldness" that characterizes the cancer-ridden body-cancer patients often complain of feeling cold, but their bodies become warmer after treatment with mistletoe.

Typically, European doctors using Iscador administer the first series of injections to observe any undesirable reactions. The medicine is injected (subcutaneously, as a serum) in the morning, several times per week. Iscador can be taken orally, either as a tincture or in homeopathic form, but only if the immune system is already 'somewhat responsive.' If one's immune system is weak or severely compromised then the injection is recommended. "The strength that we use for injecting Iscador depends on the energy reserves of the patient and how much immune reserve they have left" says Stoff. "However, all the injections are low potency."

Larix-Larch Arabinogalactan Powder, or Ara-6 A sweet-tasting medicinal powder highly concentrated in complex carbohydrates or polysaccharides (long-chain sugars) derived from the Western Larch tree (Larix occidentalis). A special property it has is its capacity for stimulating the activity of various types of immune cells. Ara-6 also dissolves in water easily and maintains its chemical stability over a wide range of concentrations, pH, and temperature changes.

Definitive results with Larix have been seen in terms of increasing natural killer (NK) cell activity. "We know that NK activity can help a person with cancer, particularly when trying to prevent new tumors or micrometastases. "Larix seems to stimulate NK activity quite well while also helping to raise the individual's energy level," states Dr Stoff. Ara-6 also has the ability to stimulate the activity of macrophages, another major part of the body's anticancer defenses, which may be just as significant as its positive effect on NK activity.

Biochemists have determined that a sugar component of Larix may stimulate NK activity in a manner similar to the sugar component of Viscum album (mistletoe).' The combination of these substances could therefore have an additive effect in terms of activating anticancer defenses. Dr. Stoff recommends taking a teaspoon in a glass of vegetable juice or water times a day. Typically people who take Ara-6 are advised to take supplemental vitamin C at the same time because it can enhance the effectiveness of Ara-6. Both of these botanicals may be acquired and administered by a qualified alternative physician of nutritionist.

The Importance of Detoxification in a Cancer Reversal Program

Most all alternative medicine doctors and holistic practitioners agree that too many toxins in the body produce illness. Signs and symptoms of the toxic body can include being overweight, bloating and intestinal gas, insomnia, nausea, bad breath, asthma, constipation, tension, headaches, depression, stress, allergies, weakness, intense menstrual discomforts and problems, and many others. Cancer patients wishing to get a head start on eliminating cancer from their body must seek a form of detoxification, which will maximize results of eliminating cancer from the body and if one is going through conventional treatment, a detoxifying program will maximize the results as well.

Many cancer patients who seek alternative treatments have already had conventional treatment and are already nutritionally depleted and overloaded with toxins. If this were the case, it would be highly dangerous to attempt a strong detoxification program. It is a delicate balance in these cases where the liver's functioning should be stimulated in a gentle and gradual way while supporting the immune system. A patient should try to ingest foods and herbs to reduce stress on a toxic organ or body region.

In the case of an overburdened liver, a botanical medicine such as Essiac is good to ingest, which has "an affinity for the liver and doesn't stress the kidneys," states Dr. Stoff. Also good to take is silymarin (milk over thistle). "This herb is valuable in helping cancer patients recover from the toxic effects of chemotherapy or heavy drug use in general. No other single herb seems to have as much detoxifying, liver-regenerating power."

Some people specify juicing and ingesting nothing but raw juice for detoxification and intense immune boosting. It is not always recommended that one drink large amounts of raw juices such as carrot juice at first, as is sometimes recommended for cancer patients, because the liver generally cannot fully convert the beta carotene in carrots to vitamin A. Small amounts, sometimes diluted with two part pure water (two parts carrot juice) is desirable in cases where the liver is not overburdened.

The effort alone to digest properly large amounts of raw juice can place an additional stress on the body. An overly toxic liver can be relieved through simple dietary changes such as avoiding oils and high-fat foods and emphasizing raw leafy greens and brightly colored vegetables. Once steps have been taken to relieve a toxic liver and one is feeling fairly well, a regimen of drinking raw juices, especially carrot and wheatgrass juice, can help the body fight cancer cells and other invading problems such as viruses.

Toxic kidneys is another condition commonly seen among cancer patients, particularly in those who have received extensive conventional treatments. If the kidneys are not functioning well, patient should be careful with supplements, such as large amounts of amino acids, minerals, and high-dose vitamin C. The reason for this is that these nutrients are all water-soluble and pass through the kidney to be eliminated through urination. Instead, one would want to take these slowly as healing is under way and under the supervision a qualified nutritionist.

In general, when the elimination system is in a toxic and not functioning well, the reason for the poor response must be determined. A toxic colon or kidney means there is elevated creatinine, constipation, gas, bloating, cramps, and often a skin rash. A heavy meat-eating diet is the number one cause particularly when coupled with a sedentary lifestyle. Starting a regular exercise program (one tailored to the specific needs of the individual and disseminated by their physician) and abstaining from eating lots of meat can make an **immediate difference**.

The colon can sometimes be stimulated to work better by checking out some substances that a nutritionist might recommend. These could include Epsom salts, taken orally, Chinese herbs (such as San She Dan), and special fiber supplements all individually determined with the help of a nutritionist, to stimulate the colon, and help it work better. There are several detoxification packages that one can purchase also. Working from below, the use a coffee enema is very effective and can be administered by a holistic health practitioner specializing in colonic irrigation therapy.

This is the only detoxifying technique some physicians working alternatively use on a routine basis with cancer patients. It is used primarily to stimulates liver detoxification.

New Pharmaceutical Substances for Treating Cancer.
Alklyglycerols (Shark Liver Oil).

A group of compounds called alkylglycerols (pronounced all-kill-gliss-ser-alls) can bolster anticancer defenses and protect the body against the harmful effects of radiation-induced injury." The richest source of these special fats (also called "ether lipids" or ("Alkyl Lyso - phospholipid") is shark liver oil, and these are found to a lesser extent in the fats found in mother's milk, which contains 10 times more alkylglycerols than cow's milk.

Animal studies have indicated that alkylglycerols have anti-tumor activity, probably mediated through certain immune cells (macrophages) in the form of direct and selective destruction to cancer cells. Cell culture studies have shown that alkylglycerols are 'selectively toxic against cancer cells" and this "selection" seems to be affected by the cholesterol concentration of the cancer cell; as the cholesterol level drops, the cancer cells die more rapidly.

Extracts of shark liver oil may help people tolerate both chemotherapy and radiation. The administration of alkylglycerols prior to radiation treatment was found to cause advanced tumors to regress toward less advanced stages; alkylglycerols also caused reversal of tumor growth in animal studies.

A possible explanation for these findings is that this substance can inhibit a variety of tumor-promoting substances, including the "bad" eicosanoids and platelet-activating factor (PAF). One potential area of concern, however, is contamination of shark liver oil by ocean pollutants. No published research that is known of has yet addressed this issue nor have the potential toxicities at normal doses been adequately studied.

Scientists at Johns Hopkins University School of medicine found that a synthetic form of **squalamine** (found in the tissues of the dogfish shark), originally derived from shark liver, is effective in controlling the growth of brain tumors in rats and in extending their lives. The substance suppresses the formation of new blood vessels in the tumor, thus preventing it from growing, reports the New York Times (May 1, 1996).

Antinioplastons.

Beginning in the 1960's, Stanislaw Burzynski, M.D., isolated several peptides (chains of amino acids, the building blocks of protein) from human urine and found them to be effective in controlling the growth of certain types of cancer. Dr. Burzynski originally identified and isolated from the urine of healthy humans, 5 different antineoplastons (meaning substances that work against [anti] a neoplasm (an abnormal growth of new tissue, such as a tumor).

He determined that these molecules have a strong anticancer effect at a genetic level: specifically, they appear to stimulate the activity of "tumor suppressor genes," genes that literally turn off the activity of certain oncogenes (genes that promote tumor growth). By this action, antineoplastons can actually stop cells from multiplying out of control, eventually producing a tumor mass, said Dr. Burzynski. It is almost as if cancer results from a deficiency of antineoplastons.

Dr. Burzynski has successfully used antineoplastons, which he produces himself in an FDA-approved manufacturing facility in his Houston, Texas', clinic. Currently, he has 65 different treatment protocols using 2 antineoplaston formulas. The protocols differ according to type and size of tumor, although best results appear to come from treating brain tumors, metastatic breast cancer, and non-Hodgkin's lymphoma.

As part of a study, he used antineoplastons to treat 20 patients who had advanced-stage astrocytoma, a particularly fast-growing type of brain tumor that tends to occur in young children. Nearly 80% of them responded favorably, and a number of them were tumor free 4 years later.At the Ninth International Symposium on Future Trends in Chemotherapy in March 1990, Dr. Dvorit Samid stated, "Antineoplaston AS2-1 profoundly inhibits oncogene expression and the proliferation of malignant cells without exhibiting any toxicity toward normal cells. 'Based on clinical results of 7 studies presented at the conference, Dr. Samid concluded: "Antineoplaston therapy restores to the body those natural compounds that have anticancer activity.

Because they are natural compounds, the body tolerates them well, and therefore we minimize the problem of adverse effects. Antineoplastons could be a very valuable,
effective, and safe approach to cancer therapy."

Carnivora.

This extract of the meat-eating plant Venus' flytrap (Dinoea muscipula) was introduced into cancer therapy by German oncologist Helmet Keller, medical director of the Chronic Disease Control and Treatment Center in Bad Steven, Germany. Dr. Keller has conducted extensive studies of the intravenous delivery of Carnivora as used in German cancer clinics.

The medicine contains one-third pressed Venus Fly Trap juice, one-third alcohol, and one-third purified water. Dr. Keller has treated over 2,000 cancer patients with Camivora, so named in honor of the plant's well-known insect-eating ability. One of the active ingredients appears to be a chemical called plumbagin which has anticancer properties;" when topically applied, it can lead to a total reversal of skin cancer."

Dr. Keller's laboratory studies indicate that Camivora directly inhibits the metabolic activity of cancer cells. In a clinical study of 210 cancer patients for whom conventional treatments had failed, each received 50-60 drops of Camivora orally 5 times a day plus one intravenous infusion daily. The results were excellent: 16% of patients showed tumor remission and 40% had no further tumor progression; in the remaining 44% no improvement was noted, although about one-quarter of these patients experienced a palliative effect. This means they felt a decrease in subjective complaints and pain and an increase in appetite, vitality, and positive attitude, according to Dr. Keller. The study showed that more than half, or 56%, experienced either a tumor remission or their cancer became more stable and did not worsen.

Camivora is an immunomodulator, which means it stimulates the activity of T helper cells. This in turn enables the body to wage a more vigorous defense against the illness, explains Dr. Keller. Carnivore appears to target tumor cells and bolster the immune system.

After the intravenous program is completed, intramuscular injections may be carried out several times a week until the treatment program is finished. People should not attempt to produce their own Camivora, however, since it first must be purified of naturally occurring plant toxins that would otherwise cause fevers and other adverse reactions. Instead, they should contact one of the alternative physicians listed below or a qualified nutritionist for more information.

Bovine Cartilage.

In 1954, John F. Prudden, M.D., discovered that bovine cartilage had a remarkable ability to help wounds heal faster. Today, bovine tracheal cartilage is one of the few substances proven to accelerate wound healing, which is why most surgical textbooks mention it. But Dr. Prudden became deeply intrigued with the wider therapeutic potential of this obscure substance. He was able to observe it dramatically shrink a breast tumor and reduce the malignant ulceration of the chest wall of a desperate patient, and he was convinced.

The development of new blood vessels (angiogenesis) is a prerequisite for tumor growth, yet this process can be stopped by cartilage from either cows or sharks. Bovine tracheal cartilage (BTC) causes a general activation of the body's anticancer defenses and has demonstrated effectiveness against cancers of the ovary, pancreas, colon, and testes; a BTC extract inhibited the growth of tumor cell lines from 22 Patients with various cancers.

Since 1972, Dr. Pradden has used BTC to successfully treat many cases of advanced cancer; the partial and complete response rate, taken overall, is approximately 30% within a 7-month treatment period.

In a what is now a classic study released in 1985, Dr. Pradden reported on the results of a trial with 31 cancer patients all of whom had failed to respond to conventional therapies or had a cancer that was not treatable at all. After starting a regimen of cartilage- typically 9 g daily, taken orally in 3 -gram installments 3 times daily, 90% of the patients had a partial or complete response.

Dr. Prudden also reports success in causing a large rectal tumor to disappear, leaving the patient cancer free for 18 years after treatment. Bovine cartilage produced a complete healing of breast cancer after all other therapies had failed; this patient remained free of cancer for IO years until her death from other causes. A man with prostatic cancer that had spread to the bones had a complete remission. An elderly woman, aged 79, with kidney cancer that had spread to her lungs and liver, survived 4 years with much improved conditions.

Strictly speaking it is not a cure because patients who respond to it must continue taking it at the rate of 9 mg. daily for the rest of their lives to avoid a possible remission. It also takes up to 4 months for the initial positive effects to show up in the system, Dr. Prudden advises. In more than 2 5 years, he has never observed any toxic side effects from using bovine cartilage, even with doses 3 times as high as the therapeutic dose.

Copyright - 2017. Published by Cancer Group Institute. www.cancergroup.com 59

Bovine cartilage also contains large sugar molecules called mucopolysaccharides that appear to block cell division n in the cancerous cells. If the cells cannot divide, they cannot multiply, which means the cancer doesn't spread. For the therapeutic dose needed, bovine cartilage if 4 times less expensive than shark cartilage and it takes approximately 70 g of shark cartilage to get healing results in contrast to 9 grams of bovine cartilage.

Other alternative pharmacological substances worth checking into which are relatively unknown except to alternative cancer physicians are Hydrazine Sulfate, a synthetic chemical which inhibits the loss of protein or body mass caused by cancer; Indocin (Indomethancin) which is a member of the family of nonsteroidal medications and growing research indicates that indocin may be effective against various cancers; Mellitin, dervived from the stinger of honeybees,; Nucleic Acids (2LC1 and 2 LCL1), which are two homeopathic blends that have been shown to be effective in advanced cancers; and 714X, a compound consisting of nitrogen-rich camphor and organic salts that seem effective against many forms of cancer. All of these must be taken under the supervision of a physician or qualified nutritionist.

Alternative Clinical Approaches.

Heat Therapy - A clinical process called hyperthermia, which is the raising of the body's temperature is another detoxification technique used with some success as part of an alternative cancer treatment program. For example, heat can be localized with the help of medical devices that direct microwaves to the tumor, raising the temperature of the tumor itself to 42' C or 43' C (1 07.6' F to 109.4' F); this procedure is particularly effective in controlling superficial tumors located on or near the skin. Conventional doctors have used this approach, known by them as diathermy, to lower the effective dosage range of radiation treatment. In the process, patients can reduce or even eliminate the need for radiation therapy. Only a relatively small rise in body temperature can make a huge difference," says Robert Atkins, M.D., who includes it in his cancer protocols.

Though the principle sounds simple, the technique is far more complicated, thanks to the body's ability to regulate its internal temperature. As any sauna enthusiast will attest, the human body likes heat only to a point. When the body temperature rises, blood flow increases to dissipate the excess heat. One way to circumvent the body's ability to regulate its temperature is to apply the heat locally, targeting a specific tumor.

This can be done with the use of microwave's and ultrasound, which can be directed at parts of the body with great precision. Ultrasound causes an increase in body temperature as a result of friction produced at the molecular level as the high-energy sound waves strike different body tissues. (For whole-body or large-area treatments, multiple ultrasound applicators may be used.) Radiant heating devices produce infrared heat that is applied to the body. Extracorporeal heating involves removing blood from the body (via plastic tubes placed into the veins), heating it, and returning it to the body at a higher temperature.

Normally, part of the damage caused by radiation is repaired by the cancer cells, enabling some to survive; however, heat foils this self-repairability. Taken together, these facts tend to make tumors more vulnerable to heat treatment than normal tissue.

At the Duke Hyperthermia Program of the Duke University Medical Center in Durham, North Carolina, considerable success has been reported in using hyperthermia to treat soft-tissue sarcomas and often-deadly recurrences of breast cancer. One recent study found that radiation combined with hyperthermia was 30% more effective against breast cancer than radiation treatment alone.

Tumors located near the surface of the body appear to be more amenable to treatment than deep-tissue tumors. "I try never to use radiation treatment - which is even more dangerous than most forms of chemotherapy-without also using hyperthermia," says Dr. Atkins. "Thanks to hyperthermia, we can shrink tumors with far less radiation today to get the same therapeutic outcome in cancer patients, and our patients' immune systems and overall health are faring much better as a result."

Hyperthermia is approved in the U.S. for treatment of breast cancer recurrence, and it is covered by insurance. This is how heat therapy works: Heat results when atoms and molecules vibrate and move around at a higher rate or frequency. The body uses its own internally generated heat to protect itself from viruses, bacteria, and other harmful substances. A fever is the body's highly evolved attempt to destroy invading organisms and to sweat impurities out through the skin. Fever is an effective natural process of curing disease and restoring health; heat therapy, or hyperthermia, represents a way to create fever to call out this natural healing process.

Cancer cells are more heat sensitive than normal tissues and are more easily killed by heating. Localizing the heat is important, since one cannot raise the whole-body temperature to 42' C or 43' C without lethal consequences.

Another strategy is to raise the whole-body temperature in a more moderate way, from 37' C to 40' C (98.6' F to 104' E). This may be performed by using whole-body wet wraps, saunas, and hot baths. When used in combination with taking ginseng or other substances that increase the effect of heat, it can be of value in cancer treatment. One may also take a hot bath with a cup of Epsom salts and a cup of baking soda mixed into the bath water, which can heat the body to a moderate degree and provide a gentle detoxifying effect.

One substance that may be combined with hyperthermia to enhance its effectiveness is the bioflavonoid quercetin. This bioflavonoid helps stop histamine release. Quercetin can inhibit the synthesis of proteins (heat shock proteins) that help tumors resist heat stress; also quercetin inhibits the transport of lactic acid out of cancer cells. By doing this, it lowers the pH inside the cancer cell, and reduces the likelihood that tumor cells will proliferate or metastasize.

Thus, the anticancer effect of quercetin in the context of hyperthermia is twofold: it makes the inside of cancer cells more acidic (lowers the intracellular pH, which helps kill the cell) and makes the cancer cells more vulnerable to the effects of heat. Dr. Stoff's typical dosage is 1000-1500 mg taken 3 times daily.

Only recently has conventional medicine caught up with this practice and begun to incorporate hyperthermia in the orthodox treatment protocols for cancer.

Exercise- To give the detoxification systems an added boost, It is frequently advised patients to engage in regular stress-free physical activities such as walking, jogging, cycling, or swimming. Gentle games with constant movement such as volleyball and basketball can help stimulate the lymphatic system and overall metabolism, thereby aiding detoxification. If one has access to a yoga class, this can be of invaluable assistance in stimulating immunity and lowering stress by movement and heating of the body without hard impact.

Exercise speeds up the neutralization and removal of poisons from the body's cells and tissues through sweating and increased urination and stimulates the activity of natural killer cells and other components of the body's anticancer defenses. When the body's temperature rises during exercise there tends to be an increase in the production of pyrogen, a substance that enhances the function of white blood cells and thus the immune function is working properly.

However, excessive exercise can be detrimental. Dr. Stoff cautions that it can produce an excess of free radicals and lactic acid, both of which tend to promote cancer. Patients should become involved in an exercise program in a gradual and sensitive manner, respecting their abilities and attitudes. "A fundamentalist Christian will often walk out of your office if you suggest they practice yoga," Dr. Stoff says. "It's important to understand where a person is coming from in their beliefs and to support them; otherwise your recommendations will likely fall on deaf ears."

Magnetic - Field Therapy.

The use of magnets and electrical devices to generate controlled magnetic fields has many medical applications and has proven to be one of the most effective means available for diagnosing human illness and disease. Clinical evidence shows that cancers, subjected to a negative magnetic field, can start to reverse as the magnetic energy helps restore oxygen levels and reduce acidity.

Electromagnetic energy is an integral part of the human body. The world is surrounded by magnetic fields: some are generated by the Earth's magnetism; others are generated by solar storms and changes in the weather. Magnetic fields are also created by everyday electrical devices: motors, televisions, office equipment, computers, electrically heated water beds, electric blankets, microwave ovens, the electrical wiring in homes, and the Power lines that supply them.

The human body produces subtle magnetic fields that are generated by the chemical reactions within the cells and the ionic currents of the nervous system. The catalytic reactions of enzymes are all driven by magnetic fields and produce magnetic fields themselves."

Recently, scientists have discovered that external magnetic fields can affect the body's functioning in both positive and negative ways, and this observation has led to the development of magnetic field therapy. The use of magnets and electrical devices to generate controlled magnetic fields has many medical applications and has proven to be one of the most effective means available for diagnosing human illness and disease.

In addition to its diagnostic power, magnetic field therapy can be used to treat physical and emotional disorders.

Magnets and electromagnetic therapy devices are now being used to relieve symptoms and reverse degenerative diseases, eliminate pain, facilitate the healing of broken bones, counter the effects of stress, and address the reversal of cancer.

In 1974, researcher Albert Roy Davis noted that positive and negative magnetic energies have different effects upon the biological systems of animals and humans. He found that magnets could be used to arrest and kill cancer cells in animals, and could also be used in the treatment of arthritis, glaucoma, infertility, and diseases related to aging. Davis concluded that negative polarity magnetic fields have a beneficial effect on living -organisms, whereas positive polarity magnetic fields have a stressful effect.

In tests to evaluate the risk to cancer patients of exposure to magnetic fields, tissue cultures were exposed to a positive magnetic field for a prolonged period. The cancer grew. With prolonged exposure to a negative magnetic field, the cancer receded.

Magnetic Field Therapy as a Primary or Adjunctive Cancer Treatment.

According to Wolfgang Ludwig, So.D., Ph.D., Director of the Institute for Biophysics in Horn, Germany, "Magnetic field therapy is a method that penetrates the whole human body and can treat every organ without chemical side effects."

At Dr. Ludwig's Institute for Biophysics, magnetic field therapy has been effective in the treatment of cancer. Robert Becker, M.D., an orthopedic surgeon and prime researcher of magnetic energy, found that weak electric currents promote the healing of broken bones.

Dr. Becker also brought national attention to the fact that electromagnetic interference from power lines and home appliances can pose a serious hazard to human health. "The scientific evidence leads to only one conclusion: The exposure of living organisms to abnormal electromagnetic fields results in significant abnormalities in physiology and function."

With Magnetic Field Therapy, Energy Changes at the Cellular Level.

There are numerous forms of magnetic field therapy, including static field magnets and pulsating magnetic fields generated by electrical devices. The magnetic fields produced by magnets or electromagnetic generating devices are able to penetrate the human body and therapeutically affect the functioning of the nervous system, organs, and cells.

According to William Philpott, M.D., a magnetic therapy pioneer of Choctaw, Oklahoma, when used properly, magnetic field therapy has no known harmful side effects. Dr. Philpott has found that the "negative magnetic field" can even reverse cancer. (A compass or magnetometer is used to identify the positive and negative magnetic poles.") "Whether it is a cut, bruise, broken bone, infection or cancer, it is the negative magnetic energy that heals," Dr. Philpott states. He also points out that the same magnetic energy is capable of countering the toxic effects of poisonous chemicals, addictive drugs, and other potentially harmful substances.

The therapy is based on the fact that the body is surrounded by a magnetic field and is composed of numerous smaller magnetic fields, which become disturbed in the course of illness. Clinical research indicates that magnetic therapy can restore the body's normal, healthy magnetic fields and thereby promote recovery from cancer, says Dr. Philpott. Positive magnetic energy possesses no capacity for regeneration or cancer reversal. The body must maintain a negative magnetic field in order for healing to occur.

The key to how magnetic fields can stimulate healing, and help in reversing cancer, has to do with its effect on oxygen, says Dr. Philpott. Magnetic fields can stimulate metabolism and increase the amount of oxygen available to cells. It has been speculated by Dr. Philpott have that oxygen deficiency, coupled with acidity, are unique characteristics of all cancer cells, and are actually the two main causes of cancer.

The more alkaline pH produced by a negative magnetic field is necessary for healing as cancer cannot grow in an alkaline environment, Dr. Philpott explains.

This common denominator is called acid-hypoxia, and refers to a cellular condition of acidity and low oxygen status. According to Dr. Philpott, cancer only develops in acid-hypoxia cellular tissue. Numerous precipitating factors, such as carcinogens, excess free radicals, maladaptive reactions to foods, geopathic stress (Earths vibrations which rise up through the Earth and are distorted by weak electromagnetic fields created by subterranean running water, certain mineral concentrations, fault lines and underground cavities.

The vibration distorted becomes abnormally high and harmful to living organisms.), aberrant electromagnetic energy, and 60-cycle per second electrical pulsing frequency, can produce acid hypoxia. This is when normal cells can turn to cancerous cells. A normal cell is alkaline, because otherwise oxygen could not be there for the cell to make its energy.

A key chemical called adenosine triphosphate (ATP) is made by cells as an energy source through the use of oxygen; it is central to the way in which energy is released and transported. This process is called oxidative phosphorylation and involves the addition of phosphate to adenosine, thereby creating high-energy phosphate bonds. Normal, healthy human cells use oxygen to produce ATP as an energy source. Oxidative phosphorylation depends on conditions of alkalinity and high levels of molecular oxygen to function properly, says Dr. Philpott.

Infectious microorganisms (bacteria, fungi, and some intestinal parasites) and cancer cells have a different way of producing energy; it is called fermentative phosphorylation. Here, under conditions of acidity and low or no oxygen, ATP is made through the fermentation of glucose (blood sugar) instead of through the use of oxygen. "In fact, if there were a lot of oxygen present, it would not work. Oxygen and the alkaline pH would inhibit this fermentation process, which requires a condition of acidity and no or low oxygen," explains Dr. Philpott.

Healthy human cells have the ability to make ATP by either method just described. However, fermentative phosphorylation cannot sustain life for humans but it will sustain the life of cancer cells, bacteria, fungi, and certain parasites. "The human bio-oxidative energy system is able to defeat the biological life energy system of cancer cells," he says.

Further, we get an estimated 10,000 injuries to our genetic material, or DNA, every day from carcinogenic chemicals. DNA can be repaired as long as the cells have plenty of oxygen and are alkaline; but if it is in an acid state it doesn't repair, and cancer cells can rapidly reproduce.

One other link involves a crucial series of enzymes. These enzymes help revert oxygen back to its normal molecular state where it can actively initiate normal oxidative phosphorylation process. A positive magnetic field blocks the catalytic function of these enzymes and without sufficient negative magnetic energy acting as a kind of energy nutrient, the enzymes can't function to reverse conditions leading to cancer. "Thus, in addition to acid-hypoxia (oxygen shortage in acid conditions), a lack of negative magnetic energy can also be considered a major cause of cancer," Dr. Philpott states.

To defeat cancer, the cellular conditions must be changed so cancer cannot exist. Thus, the alkalinity and oxygen level in the cells must be raised with a negative magnetic field. A negative magnetic field applied to the human body has an amazing ability to remove cancerous conditions and replace them with an oxygen rich environment where cancer cells can't survive.

Magnetic field therapy can reduce the side effects of chemotherapy, and as previously mentioned positively influences the activity of enzymes. The negative magnetic field energy activates the oxidoreductase system, which is a highly efficient enzyme system that aids in detoxification. According to Dr. Philpott, "These systems turn harmful toxic acids into harmless and biologically necessary alkali substances. This then provides body cells with an abundance of necessary molecular oxygen for biological energy production."

Clinical Guidelines for Treating Cancers with Magnetic Therapy.

The guidelines for treatment with this therapy require a physician's diagnosis and monitoring under the supervision of a Scientific Institutional Publication Board. This therapy has been approved by the FDA and based on toxicity studies are classified as "not essentially harmful." Magnetic therapy for cancer continues to be considered experimental and warrants more studies. The indication is however, that a negative magnetic field has been observed in both animals and humans to reverse cancer lesions.

Dangerous, Disease Causing Food Ingredients To Avoid.

High-Fructose Corn Syrup - The Corn Refiners Association recently asked the FDA in the U.S. to allow high-fructose corn syrup (HFCS) to be renamed 'corn sugar' for labelling purposes. In Canada, the product is labelled as glucose/fructose and is found in an alarmingly wide array of products, from yogurt to bread to lunch meats. Some scientists say HFCS is more dangerous than regular sugar because it can affect normal appetite and can contain mercury

Gluten - Sufferers of celiac disease have long avoided this substance, which is found in almost any product made from wheat, oats, barley or rye, but now many who don't test positive for the disease are identifying as **'gluten intolerant'** and going **'G-Free.'** Gastro-intestinal problems are the most common symptom of gluten intolerance

Food Coloring - While many parents blame sugar for their children's hyperactivity, it may be the food coloring that is to blame. Recent studies suggest that artificial coloring agents found in everything from candy to sausages aggravate attention-deficit disorder and attention-deficit hyperactivity disorder. Several studies have even shown that academic performance increases in schools where artificial ingredients, including colorings, are banned.

Nitrates and Nitrites - Many recent studies have linked processed meats to heart disease and cancer and nitrates and nitrites may be the key. Found in hot dogs, bacon, deli meats and other prepared meats, the preservatives can form carcinogenic compounds called nitrosamines when heated. These nitrosamines can contribute to the formation of brain cancers and leukemia

Flour - Not all flours are bad for you, but the highly refined white flour found in many breads may be detrimental to your health. Often produced using chlorine and peroxides, the product emerges without its original nutrients. The body processes the flour as sugar, contributing to the epidemics of obesity and diabetes

Ractopamine - Approved for use in Canada, ractopamine is a chemical used to make pigs grow more quickly as they approach slaughter.

Consequently, levels of the chemical have little time to be processed and can remain at high levels in the eventual product. Ractopamine poses particular danger to those with heart conditions. The product has already been banned by more than 100 countries

---

Following is a list from "An Alternative Medicine Definitive Guide to Cancer" by W. John Diamond, M.D. of Alternative cancer physicians. Much of the alternative information for this publication has been found in his book.

Robert C. Adkins, M.D.
The Atkins Center, 152 East 55th St.
New York, NY 10022
tel: 212-758-2110

W. John Diamond, M.D.
Triad Medical Center
4600 Kietzke Lane
M-242, Reno, NV 89502
tel: 702-829-2277

Steven B. Edelson, M.D.
3833 Roswell Rd, Ste. 110
Atlanta, GA 30342

Keith Block, M.D.
Block Medical Center
1800 Sherman Ave.
Ste. 515, Evanston, IL 60201
tel: 847-492-3040

Douglas Brodie, M.D.
309 Kirman Ave, #2
Reno, NV 89502
tel: 702-324-7071

Patrick Donovan, M.D.
University Health Clinic
5312 Roosevelt Way NE

tel: 404-841-0088

Tori Hudson, N.D.
A Woman's Time Natural
Medicine
2067 N.W. Lovejoy
Portland, OR 97209
tel: 503-222-0276

Victor A. Marcial-Vega, M.D.
4037 Poinciana Ave.
Coconut Grove, FL 33133
tel: 305-442-1233

Emanuel Revici, M.D., Ken Korins
M.D.
The Revici Life Science Center, Inc.
200 W. 57th St. Ste. 402
New York, NY 10019
tel: 212-246-5122

Geronimo Rubio, M.D.
American Metabolic Institute
555 Saturn Blvd. Bldg B M/S 432
San Diego, CA 92154
tel: 619-267-1107

Charles B. Simone, M.MS., M.D.
Simone Protective Cancer Ctr
123 Franklin Corner Rd.
Lawrenceville, NJ 08648
tel: 609-896-2646

Jesse Stoff, M.D.
Solstice Clinical Associates
2122 N. Craycroft Road, #112

Seattle, WA 98105
tel: 206-525-8015

James W. Forsythe, M.D., H.M.D.
Cancer Screening and Treatment
Center
75 Pringle Way, Ste. 909
Reno, NV 89502
tel: 702-329-5000

Dan Labriola, N.D.
P.O. Box 99157
Seattle, WA 98199
tel: 206-285-4993

Martin Milner, M.D.
Center For Natural Medicine, Inc.
1330 SE 39th Ave.
Portland, OR 97214
tel: 503-232-1100

Robert C. Rountree, M.D.
Helios Health Center
4150 Darley Ave. Ste. 1
Boulder, CO 80303
tel: 303-499-9224

Michael B. Schachter, M.D.
Schachter Ctr For Complementary
Medicine
Two Executive Blvd., Ste. 202
Suffern, NY 10901
tel: 914-368-4700

Vincent Speckhart, M.D., M.D.H.
902 Graydon Ave, No 2
Norfolk, VA 23507

Tucson, AZ 85712
tel: 520-290-4516

Lawrence H. Taylor, M.D.
Advanced Medicine Center
1000 Cordova Court
Chula Vista, CA 91910
tel: 888-422-7434

International Listings

Ernesto R. Contreras, M.D.
Oasis Hospital, Tijuana No. 19
Apartado Postal No. 179
Playas de Tijuana, B.C. 22700
Mexico
tel: 5266-80-18 U.S 800-700-1850

Abram Hoffer, M.D. Ph.D.
2727 Quadra, Ste. 3
Victoria, British Columbia
Canada, V8T 4E5
tel: 250-386-8156

tel: 804-622-0014

Jack O. Taylor, M.S., D.C.
Dr. Taylor's Wellness Center, Inc.
3601 Algonquin Rd., Ste. 801
Rolling Meadows, IL 60008
tel: 847-222-1192

Etienne Callebout, M.D.
10 Harley Street
London, England W1N1AA
tel: 44-171-467-8300

Meridian Energy Therapies (METs) became a separate healing field when a US psychologist, Dr Roger Callahan, began to use insights about the body's energy system to treat psychological problems with astonishing success in the early 1980s.

A large part of METs is still devoted to treating psychological problems such as fear, phobias, anxieties, motivation problems etc. This is also known as "Energy Psychology" and this rapidly developing field is re-writing the definitions of what is causing mental disturbances and how to treat such disturbances swiftly, gently and very effectively.

Copyright - 2017. Published by Cancer Group Institute. www.cancergroup.com 73

Originally, there were only a few separate techniques. But in recent years, active research and feedback by a large number of innovators who came from other fields of human healing and found in the new Meridian Energy Therapies answers and routes of enquiry that were simply not available before has created a wonderful variety of METs.

The following Members have been certified by the **Association for Meridian Energy Therapies** (The AMT) as Meridian Energy Therapy Practitioners. This qualification also includes intensive knowledge of Emotional Freedom Techniques (EFT).

Sebnem Akalin. Istanbul, Turkey. Cell # 90 530 517 75 40

Ilknur Akarsu. Turkey. Phone +90 532 495 76 18

Fatime Akgöz. Izmir, Turkey. Phone +90 505 708 95 55

Cigdem Akin. Istanbul, Turkey. Phone 0533 308 23 82

Nazmiye Akyıldız. Istanbul, Turkey. Phone +90 505 400 94 36

Aynur Apaydin. İstanbul, Turkey. Phone 0 532 733 31 05

Karen Aquinas. Oregon, United States. www.biofieldhealthservices.com

Gulcan Arpacioglu Adams. Istanbul, Turkey. Phone 902163023865 or Cell # 532 503 1776

Cagatay Atasagun. Istanbul, Turkey. Phone 0533 337 4444

Murat Aydın. Kayseri, Turkey. Phone +90 533 657 3297

GÜl Aytekİn Özen. İstanbul, Turkey. Phone 90 533 248 30 15

Alan Balfour. West Yorkshire, England. Phone 0113 2585438

Mathilde Barbier. Surrey, England. Phone (44) 07947 319 362

Tina Beckham. Kent, England. Ashford, Kent, England

Wendy Leanne Beresford. Gloucestershire, England. Phone 07855699463

Jacqueline Besseling. Nederland. Prof. Evertslaan 130b. 2628 XZ Delft. 06

125 843 48 or E-mail: jacqueline.besseling@gmail.com

Wendy Birse. Perth and Kinross, Scotland. Cell # 07774 813 178

Arzu Bıyıklı. Ataşehir, Turkey. Phone +90 533 322 19 78

Joanne Blachut. Queensland, Australia.

https://joanneblachut.goe.ac/contact/

Shiloh Blachut. Queensland, Australia.

https://shilohblachut.goe.ac/contact/

Gisèle Bourgoin. Québec, Canada. Phone 418-651-5938

Susan Browne. Co. Kerry, Ireland. Phone 00353 863381850

Joyce Bunton. Glasgow, Scotland. Phone 07939 984 602.

Copyright - 2017. Published by Cancer Group Institute. www.cancergroup.com 75

Stephen Carter. Maryland, United States. Phone 1-804-677-6772

Maria Chappell. South Yorkshire, England. Phone 07971 463324

Vivian Choi. Cambridgeshire, England. https://vivianchoi.goe.ac/contact/

Toks Coker. London, England. Phone 07973210107

Ber Collins. County Clare, Ireland. Phone 00353868103342

Mikael Cormont. Paris, France. Cell # 33 (0)6 27 46 01 10

Natalie Cowell. East Sussex, England. Phone 01273562649 or

Cell # 07811378087

Paula Cowell. West Sussex, England. Cell # 07919 201640

Ina Maria D'Costa. Swindon, England. Phone 01793 850499

Patricia Dancing-Elk-Walls. Texas, United States.

https://patriciadancingelk-walls.goe.ac/contact/

http://patriciawalls.net/

Grace DaSilva-Hill. Kent, England. Cell # 07590524795

Tanya Davies. Queensland, Australia. Phone 0420502722

Clare Davison. West Sussex, England. Phone 01403 734 930

Nanouschka de Wilde. Manchester, England. Phone 0161 799 6700 or Cell # 07708028278

Janet Deane. County Donegal, Ireland. https://janetdeane.goe.ac/contact/

Esen Dedeoglu. İzmir, Turkey. Phone +90 5334599781

Fiona Dilston. Edinburgh City, Scotland. Phone 07753505292

Peter Donn. Hertfordshire, England. Phone 01923 260 050

Hayley Driscoll. Cardiff, Wales. Phone 07949327385

Paula Duarte. London, England. Cell # 07845037563

Fatma El Sayed. Cairo, Egypt. Phone +20(0)1111 821271 or Cell # 2(0)1111821271

Rania El Tahtawy. Cairo, Egypt. Cell # 201097098047

Mariam Emara. Cairo, Egypt. Phone +20 10 985 97003

Sabiha Erdinc. Marmaris, Turkey. Phone +90252 4171200 or Cell # +905383660634

Gülüm Erdinç. Istanbul, Turkey. Phone +90 536 233 24 28

Berat Yeliz Eren. İstanbul, Turkey. Phone +90 533 272 57 12

Hayriye Erhan. Kayseri, Turkey. Phone +90 (0)541 243 4812

Tansu Erkan. Istanbul, Turkey. Phone 0535 358 81 65

Saliha Eroglu. Turkey, Turkey. Phone 90 532 423 15 72 or Cell #

905433304923

Naglaa Ezzat. Cairo, Egypt. Phone +20(0)1110505566

Lidia Ferreira. São Domingos De Rana, Cascais, Portugal.

https://lidiaferreira.goe.ac/contact/

Lorna Firth. Paphos, Cyprus. Phone +357 26934319 or

Cell # +357 99479426

Nelle Flynn. New South Wales, Australia. Phone +61 266777509

Davide Focardi. Co. Kildare, Ireland. Phone +353 87 6229714

Margarita Foley. Dublin, Ireland. Phone 00353863553981

Amanda Freeman. VIC, Australia. Phone 0438 668 688 or

Cell # 0438 668 688

Françoise Gins. Oxfordshire, England. Cell # 07958 131132

Philip Gowler. Berkshire, England. philgowler.co.uk.

https://philipgowler.goe.ac/contact/

Caner Gözütok. Adana, Turkey. Phone +90 532 356 58 08

Hülya Gürsözer Coşğun. Istanbul, Turkey. Phone 90 533 486 50 24

Funda Haberal. Istanbul, Turkey. Phone 05423417773

Silvia Hartmann. East Sussex, England. silviahartmann.com -

https://energyart.uk/

Saziye Hayat Etingu. Istanbul, Turkey. Phone 0216 350 01 21 or

Cell # 0533 551 51 45

Sandra Hillawi. Hampshire, England. Phone +44 (0)2392 433 928 or

Cell # 07884 443 708

Marion Hind. Northamptonshire, England. Cell # 07432 617491

Nicola Hok. London, England. Phone +44 (0)7415 88 99 63

Michaela Hope. Hampshire, England. Phone 07982 838460 or

Cell # 07982 838460

Sevil İlgün. Istanbul, Turkey. Phone +90 553 612 71 73

Kirsten Ivatts. Derbyshire, England. Phone 01335 390638 or

Cell # 07805 925275

Denise Jacques. County Durham, England.

https://denisejacques.goe.ac/contact/

Copyright - 2017. Published by Cancer Group Institute. www.cancergroup.com

Ferris Jay. County Leitrim, Ireland. Cell # 00 353 89 4171388

Katerina Kalchenko. Ukraine, Ukraine. https://happykaterina.com/ or

https://katerinakalchenko.goe.ac/contact/

Nesrin Kandemir. Istanbul, Turkey. Phone +90 532 220 44 62

Gülsun Kemaloğlu. Istanbul, Turkey. Phone +90 541 668 92 77 or

Cell # 90 541 6689277

Susan Kennard. East Sussex, England. Phone 07737100254 or

Cell # 01424715631

Aisling Killoran. Dublin, Ireland. Phone 01 2986507 or

Cell # 087 1352 122

Silvia King. East Sussex, England. https://silviaking.goe.ac/contact/

Aysun Kıran. Istanbul, Turkey. Phone +90 545 769 51 35 or

Cell # 05539457677

Dilek Kirikkanat. Turkey, Turkey. Phone 0507 245 9785 or

Cell # 00905302306226

Şebnem Koral. Bursa, Turkey. https://sebnemkoral.goe.ac/contact/

Irene Lambert. Derbyshire, England. Phone +44 (0)1332 863 290 or

Cell # 07903 711 079

Agnes Lau. Singapore, Singapore. http://www.mindtransformations.com/ or https://agneslau.goe.ac/contact/

Kym Lawn. Queensland, Australia. Phone 0406 182 735 or Cell # 0406 182 735

Isaac Lim. Selangor, Malaysia. http://www.eftwonder.com/ or https://isaaclim.goe.ac/contact/

Maria LiPuma. Oregon, United States. http://www.noble-being.com/

Irene Loudon. England. Phone 01413328829

Teresa Lynch. New Jersey, United States. Phone 908.431.0092

Katherine Lynch. New Jersey, United States. Phone 908-904-4657

Yvonne Maclean. Surrey, England. Phone 07814619265

Ray Manning. Dublin, Ireland. Phone 00353-1- 298 6507 or Cell # 00353 87 677 8049

Denise Marchisotto. New Jersey, United States. Cell # 732.718.1818

Kelly Mayne. England. Phone 07879332394

Helen McCrarren. Monaghan, Ireland.

http://www.mindbodyenergymatters.ie/ or

https://helenmccrarren.goe.ac/contact/

Siadbh McGivern. West Cork, Ireland. Phone 00353 876104498

Bridin McKenna UKCP Reg. Clinical Psychotherapist. Belfast, Northern

Ireland. Phone 07706705814 or

https://bridinmckenna.goe.ac/contact/

Michael Millett. Lincolnshire, England. Phone 01476 568800 or

Cell # 0845 6588220

Laura Moberg. New Hampshire, United States. Cell # 1 (603) 359-4782

Sharon Moore. New Jersey, United States. Phone 609-937-0502

Patricia Moreby. Warwickshire, England. Cell # 07977 099027

Tracy Morrow. Berkshire, England. Phone 01635 44200 or

Cell # 07967 340479

Auk Murat. Jawa Barat, Indonesia. Phone +6281802177777

Prabha Nagaraja. Delhi, India. https://twitter.com/@PrabNag

Karen Neil. County Durham, England. Cell # 0774 7831 850

Özlem Öğüç. Istanbul, Turkey. Phone +90 532 227 13 81

Cumasiye Ozgur. İzmir, Turkey. Phone +905303869748

Erkan Özkan. Istanbul, Turkey. Phone +90 554 958 16 44

Nimet Özkan. Istanbul, Turkey. Phone 90 554 958 16 47 or

Cell # 05549581647

Alexandra Paulino. Portugal, Portugal. Phone +351 96 610 7832 or

Cell # 96 610 78 32

António Rebocho. Lisboa, Portugal. Phone 351 933 375 724

Aleksandra Rechtman. London, England. Phone 07920746442

Eric Robins. California, United States. Phone 310 872 7446

Jonah Robins. California, United States. Phone 310 987 8874

Seda Rodop Soran. Istanbul, Turkey. Phone 0090 (212) 296 0008

Gizela Rodrigues. Lisboa, Portugal. Phone +351 965 806 862 or

Cell # 96 580 68 62

Lauren Rosenberg. London, England. Phone 07966268148

Helen Ryle. Co. Kerry, Ireland. Phone 00353 87 773 4914

Iman Saad. Cairo, Egypt. Cell # 01005838109

Copyright - 2017. Published by Cancer Group Institute. www.cancergroup.com 83

Sevgi Şahin. Istanbul, Turkey. Phone 90 0532 262 95 08 or

Cell # 0905322629508

Barbara Saph. Hampshire, England. Phone 02380 663 658 or

Cell # 07919 162 542

Heidi Saputelli. Beinwil am See, Switzerland. Phone 062 772 02 34 or

Cell # 079 578 81 08

Gamze Sari. Merkez Yalova, Turkey. Phone +905330282844

İpek Şekerdil. İzmir, Turkey. Phone +90 507 866 05 89

Sevim Sanem Selametoglu Ozcan. Antalya, Turkey.

Cell # 00905071767606

Keren Shamay. Texas, United States. Phone 1-682-233-1412

Sandra Smith. County Dublin, Ireland. Phone 00353 -86-3130969

Sadullah Sönmez. Kayseri, Turkey. Phone +90 535 270 7794 or

Cell # 905352707794

Eliezer Spetter. Jerusalem, Israel. Phone +972 29 943 704 or

Cell # 00 972 545 340 155

John Staples. Maryland, United States. Phone 703-283-5177

Dave Stewart. Greater Manchester, England. Phone 01616219653 or

Cell # 07766487194

Şengül Sürmen. Istanbul, Turkey. Phone 90 533 743 15 81

Evgenia Sverbikhina. FL, United States.

https://evgeniasverbikhina.goe.ac/contact/ or

https://evgeniasverbikhina.goe.ac/contact/

Emel Talay. İzmir, Turkey. Phone +90 532 367 04 58

Sam Thorpe. East Sussex, England. https://samcoxthorpe.goe.ac/contact/

or http://www.conscioushealthpractice.com/

Filiz Topaçlıoğlu. Ankara, Turkey. Phone +90 555 997 97 07

Sally Topham. Norfolk, England. Phone 020 7604 3619

Janine Turner. Kent, England. https://janineturner.goe.ac/contact/

Jamesylvester Urama. Nigeria. Phone 07405223058

Emmy Vadnais. Minnesota, United States. Phone 651-292-9938

Jorge Vence. Hampshire, England. Phone 07914016397 or

Cell # 07914016397

Nanette L Waller. Oklahoma, United States. Phone 918 682 6941

Ilka Wandel. Alicante, Spain. https://ilkawandel.goe.ac/contact/

Barney Wee. Singapore, Singapore. Phone +65 9667 8696

Deborah Wiggins-Hay. Herefordshire, England. Phone 07875751890 or

Cell # 07875751890

Donna Wirth. Pennsylvania, United States. Cell # 724-516-0583

Reto Wyss. Berne, Switzerland. Phone +41 62 962 9212

Aysenur Yabanigul. Istanbul, Turkey.

https://aysenuryabanigul.goe.ac/contact/

Eda Yaman. Adana, Turkey. Phone +90 543 717 22 87

Gülbahar Yeni. Turkey, Turkey. Phone +90(0) 232 336 6445 or

Cell # +90(0)532 665 5980

Beyza Yücel. Kayseri, Turkey. Phone +90 (0)532 428 0172

Ahmad Zabihi. Tehran, Iran. Phone +989121719046 or

Cell # 0757 0066556

Suzanne Zacharia. Kent, England. Phone 07533636939 or

Cell # 07533636939

Daniela Ziehn. Wesel, Germany. Phone 00492814607472 or

Poly MVA:- is a new, nontoxic, powerful antioxidant formula that **protects** both cellular DNA and RNA.

The scientifically designed mechanism of action is to "fix the cell" and control the cancer, rather than "fight the cancer" and poison the system as noted above.

Poly MVA offers an extremely powerful alternative cancer treatment without the toxic side effects associated with most Conventional Cancer Treatments.

Doctors (See Practioners List below) and **Patients worldwide** are reporting the benefits of **Poly MVA** when used as a stand-alone option or when used in conjunction with Chemotherapy and Radiation.

POLY MVA has been scientifically designed to **CORRECT DNA BREAKDOWNS** and return the damaged cells to normal cellular function.

This product was developed by **Dr. Merrill Garnett**, a highly regarded biochemist, who has been conducting research with the objective of creating an electronic frequency specificity to restore the DNA exchange energy pathway.

Poly-MVA(LAPd) compounds transfer current inward from the cell membrane phospholipid to DNA via the mitochondria.

This high flux state of inward pulsed current maintains normal electron oxygen transport, but can be shown to electrically dissociate (breakdown) membranes of primitive anaerobic (CANCER) cells including amoeba, yeasts, and certain tumors.

ALABAMA

Larry D. Brock, MD
Regenerative Medicine Center
5901 Airport Blvd. Suite E. Mobile, Alabama 36608-3156
Ph:251-342-0505
Fax: 251-342-0360
email: drbrock@regenerativemedicine-al.com
Website: www.bioidenticalhormonemd.com

ALASKA

Gary Geraly, M.D.
615 East 82nd Ave., Suite 300
Anchorage, Alaska, 99518
Phone: (907)-344-7775
Fax: (907)-522-3114
E-Mail: compmed@alaska.net

ARIZONA

Robert Zieve, MD
EuroMed Foundation
34975 N. North Valley Parkway
Bldg. 6, Suite 138
Phoenix, Arizona 85086
Phone: 602-404-0400
Fax: 602-404-0403

Website: www.euro-med.us

Harvey Abrams, DC
Rehabilitation Chiropractic Care
801 S. Power Road #107
Mesa, AZ 85206
Phone: 480-396-4400
Fax: 480-218-9324
Website: http://rehabchiro.com
Email: drabrams@rehabchiro.com

Martha Grout, MD, MD(H)
Arizona Center for Advanced Medicine
9328 E. Raintree Drive
Scottsdale, AZ 85260
Phone: (480)-240-2600
E-Mail: drmartha@arizonaadvancedmedicine.com

Charles H. Baughman, MD
Baughman & Associates Age Management Medicine
1366 N. 94th Dr. Suite E1
Peoria, AZ 85381
Phone: 623-977-0955
Fax: 623-977-3729
E-mail: crsgsdoc@cox.net
Website: www.growyounger.us

Ronald Peters, MD
MindBody Medicine Center
13951 N. Scottsdale Road
Scottsdale, AZ 85254
Phone: (480) 607-7999

Dean Silver, MD

7420 Pinnacle Road Suite 126
Scottsdale, AZ 85255
Phone: (480) 860-0689
Website: www.deansilvermd.com

CALIFORNIA

Antonio Jimenez, MD
Hope 4 Cancer Institute
13910 Lyons Valley Road, Suite L
Jamul, CA 91935
Phone: 855-366-4673
Fax: 619-956-7071
Website: www.h4cmedical.com
Email: info@h4cmedical.com

Ron Rothenberg, MD
California Healthspan Institute
320 Santa Fe Dr, #211, Encinitas, CA 92024
Phone: (760) 635-1996

Shivinder Deol, MD (Diplomate, Anti-Aging Medicine)
Anti-Aging & Wellness Center
4000 Stockdale Hwy., Suite D
Bakersfield, CA 93309
Phone: (661) 325-7452
Fax: (661) 325-7456
E-mail: doc@drdeol.com
Website: www.drdeol.com

Areas of specialty: Alternative and complementary medicine, IV vitamin C, hyberbaric oxygen, pH balance, Poly-MVA and more.

James L. Padilla, D.C.

San Diego Spine and Wellness Center
12070 Carmel Mtn. Rd. Ste. 290
San Diego, CA 92128
Phone: (858)676-1166
E-Mail: Linda@DrJamesPadilla.com
Website: http://www.DrJamesPadilla.com

Mezia O. Azinge-Obasi, MD
Doctor Paul Memorial Medical Center, Inc.
3450 W. 43rd Street, Suite 106
Los Angeles, CA. 90008
Phone: (323)290-2832
Fax: (323)290-2836
E-mail: dr.paul@dslextreme.com
Website: www.dromd.com
Areas of specialty: Care of the under-served, integrating Anti-Aging
Medicine and Alternative Medicine with Conventional Family Medicine to
achieve affordable balanced health. These include common Herbs,
Vitamins, Minerals, Hormones, pH balance, attention to blood type
differences, eating habits and more.

William S. Eidelman, MD
The Center For Healing & Transformation
(Programs for Healing Serious Illnesses)
1654 N. Cahuenga Blvd.
Los Angeles, CA 90028
Phone: 323-463-3295
Fax: 323-463-3740
E-mail: williameidelman@gmail.com
Websites: www.DrEidelman.com

Dr. Kristine Reese
LotusRain Naturopathic Clinic
5210 Balboa Ave Ste F

San Diego, CA 92117
Phone: 619-239-5433
Website: hwww.lotusrainclinic.com/

Gary Foresman, MD
Middle Path Medicine
180 W. LePoint Street Unit A
Arroyo Grande, CA 93420
Phone: (805) 481-3442
Website: www.middlepathmedicine.com

Brent Hill, DC
Hill Center for Integrated Medicine
3609 Oakdale Rd., Suite 5
Modesto, CA 95357
Phone: (209) 551-8888
Website: www.hillwellness.com/

Paul Han Soo Kim, MD
Previ Medical Group
1776 Ygnacio Valley Rd., Suite 204
Walnut Creek, CA 94598
Phone: 925-691-7546
Website: www.previmedicalgroup.com/index.html

Leigh Erin Connealy, MD
Cancer Center for Healing
6 Hughes, Suite 120B
Irvine, CA 92618
Phone: 949-581-HOPE (4673)
E-mail: info@cancercenterforhealing.com
Website: www.cancercenterforhealing.com

Area of specialty: Targeted cancer therapies including IPTLD, high-dose vitamin C, hyperbaric oxygen therapy, ultraviolet blood irradiation, light beam generator, nutraceuticals, surgery, emotional therapies and more.

CALIFORNIA
Antonio Jimenez, MD
Hope 4 Cancer Institute
13910 Lyons Valley Road, Suite L
Jamul, CA 91935
Phone: 855-366-4673
Fax: 619-956-7071
Website: www.h4cmedical.com
Email: info@h4cmedical.com

Ron Rothenberg, MD
California Healthspan Institute
320 Santa Fe Dr, #211, Encinitas, CA 92024
Phone: (760) 635-1996

Shivinder Deol, MD (Diplomate, Anti-Aging Medicine)
Anti-Aging & Wellness Center
4000 Stockdale Hwy., Suite D
Bakersfield, CA 93309
Phone: (661) 325-7452
Fax: (661) 325-7456
E-mail: doc@drdeol.com
Website: www.drdeol.com

Areas of specialty: Alternative and complementary medicine, IV vitamin C, hyberbaric oxygen, pH balance, Poly-MVA and more.

James L. Padilla, D.C.
San Diego Spine and Wellness Center

12070 Carmel Mtn. Rd. Ste. 290
San Diego, CA 92128
Phone: (858)676-1166
E-Mail: Linda@DrJamesPadilla.com
Website: http://www.DrJamesPadilla.com

Mezia O. Azinge-Obasi, MD
Doctor Paul Memorial Medical Center, Inc.
3450 W. 43rd Street, Suite 106
Los Angeles, CA. 90008
Phone: (323)290-2832
Fax: (323)290-2836
E-mail: dr.paul@dslextreme.com
Website: www.dromd.com

Areas of specialty: Care of the under-served, integrating Anti-Aging
Medicine and Alternative Medicine with Conventional Family Medicine to
achieve affordable balanced health. These include common Herbs,
Vitamins, Minerals, Hormones, pH balance, attention to blood type
differences, eating habits and more.

William S. Eidelman, MD
The Center For Healing & Transformation
(Programs for Healing Serious Illnesses)
1654 N. Cahuenga Blvd.
Los Angeles, CA 90028
Phone: 323-463-3295
Fax: 323-463-3740
E-mail: williameidelman@gmail.com
Websites: www.DrEidelman.com

Dr. Kristine Reese
LotusRain Naturopathic Clinic
5210 Balboa Ave Ste F

San Diego, CA 92117
Phone: 619-239-5433
Website: hwww.lotusrainclinic.com/

Gary Foresman, MD
Middle Path Medicine
180 W. LePoint Street Unit A
Arroyo Grande, CA 93420
Phone: (805) 481-3442
Website: www.middlepathmedicine.com

Brent Hill, DC
Hill Center for Integrated Medicine
3609 Oakdale Rd., Suite 5
Modesto, CA 95357
Phone: (209) 551-8888
Website: www.hillwellness.com/

Paul Han Soo Kim, MD
Previ Medical Group
1776 Ygnacio Valley Rd., Suite 204
Walnut Creek, CA 94598
Phone: 925-691-7546
Website: www.previmedicalgroup.com/index.html

Leigh Erin Connealy, MD
Cancer Center for Healing
6 Hughes, Suite 120B
Irvine, CA 92618
Phone: 949-581-HOPE (4673)
E-mail: info@cancercenterforhealing.com
Website: www.cancercenterforhealing.com

Area of specialty: Targeted cancer therapies including IPTLD, high-dose vitamin C, hyperbaric oxygen therapy, ultraviolet blood irradiation, light beam generator, nutraceuticals, surgery, emotional therapies and more.

COLORADO

Jonathan Singer, DO
8400 East Prentice Avenue, Suite 301
Greenwood Village, CO 80111
Phone: (303) 488-0034
Fax: (303) 488-0040
E-Mail: singerdo@aol.com
Website: www.denver-doctor.com

Johanne Wayne CN
Clinical Nutritionist
5762 W. Asbury Pl.
Lakewood, CO 80227
Tel: 303-916-5460
Fax: 303-484-6445
Email: johannewaynecn@live.com

Areas of specialty: Functional diagnostic nutrition & metabolic typing advisor level II

Brandon Lundell, DC Dipl Ac
619 Pratt St.
Longmont, CO 80501
Phone: (720) 771-0402
Fax: (303) 776-9272
E-mail: brandonlundell@juno.com

Roger Billica, MD
2362 East Prospect
Fort Collins, CO 80525
Phone: (970) 495-0999
Fax: (970) 495-1016
E-mail: trilifehealth@gmail.com or Website: www.trilifehealth.com/

CONNETICUT

Stephen T. Sinatra, M.D., F.A.C.C.,
New England Heart Center
483 West Middle Tpke,
Manchester, CT 06040
Phone: (860) 643-5101
Fax: (860) 533-9747
Website: www.drsinatra.com

Dr. Nicholas J. Palermo, D.O.
257 East Center Street
Manchester, CT 06040
Phone: (860) 645-3927
Fax: (860) 643-2531
Email: DoctorPalermo@cox.net

Yvette Whitton, ND
Adonai Optimal Health and Wellness
31 Hawleyville Road
Newton, CT 06470
Phone: 888-655-8489

DELAWARE

Gertie Hillman, R.N.
Nutrition The Way To Life
412 E. Savannah
Lewes, Delaware 11958
(302) 645-1696
Fax: (302) 645-4940
E-Mail: gerties.nutrition@verizon.net
(R.N. Hillman is a Certified Nutritionist and Herbalist and uses Poly-MVA in her Holistic Nutrition Counseling)

FLORIDA

Jeffrey Mueller, MD
Whole Family Healthcare
1201 Louisiana Ave.
Ste. E
Winter Park, Florida 32792
Phone: (407) 644-2990
Fax: (407) 644-4370
Email: Reception@WholeFamilyHealthcare.com

Area of specialty: Whole Family Healthcare also features an unrivaled program for improving the quality of life in cancer patients and in those with virtually any chronic disease, with a special emphasis on improving nutrition and digestive issues.

This comprehensive, holistic clinic offers an intensive focus on lifestyle and dietary changes, Acupuncture, computerized health screenings, Chiropractic care, Qi Gong, massage therapy, Brain maps and Neurofeedback, a large natural pharmacy, and much more.
Martin Dayton, D.O., M.D.
Dayton Medica Ctr/Office

18600 Collins Avenue
Sunny Isles Beach, Florida 33160
Phone: (305) 931-8484
Email: drdayton@daytonmedical.com
Website: www.daytonmedical.com

John Monhollon, MD
Florida Integrative Medical Center
2415 University Parkway
Sarasota, FL 34243
Phone: (941) 955-6220
Website: www.floridaintegrative.com
Areas of specialty: Acupuncture, IV Therapy, Immune and Nutritional
Support, Holistic Dentistry and more.

Gene Wei, DOM, AP
Center for Acupuncture and Integrative Medicine
668 N. Orlando Avenue #1018
Maitland, FL 32751
Phone: (407) 622-8008
Website: www.caimedicine.com

Tammy Bennett, Doctor of Oriental Medicine
Susan Chapman, ARNP
Suma Wellness Centers
212 West Bay Avenue
Longwood, FL 34750
Phone: (407) 265-1888
Fax: (407) 265-9581
Email: tammy@longwoodhealingcenter.com
Website: www.sumawellness.com

Areas of specialty: Acupuncture, anti-aging medicine, functional medicine and nutrition for cancer patients, bioidentical hormone therapy, holistic pain management for cancer patients.

GEORGIA
Nancy C. Farley, PhD
(Psychologist & Cancer Survivor)
625 Lexington Way
Woodstock, GA 30189
Phone: (770) 592-8775
E-mail: nfhaven@attbi.com

Veronique Desaulniers, DC
10863 Big Canoe
Jasper, GA 30143
Phone: (706) 579-2257
Website: www.breastcancerconqueror.com

HAWAII
Ryan Ferchoff ND
The Natural Wellness Center
Naturopathic Physician
2752 Woodlawn Drive 5-110
Honolulu, HI 96822
Phone: (808)-988-0800
E-mail: INFO@TNWC.co
Website: www.thenaturalwellnesscenter.com

Areas of specialty: Wellness Retreat In-Patient Programs and Integrative Care, IV Therapies, Naturopathic Hospital, Cancer Support Programs and Treatments.

IDAHO

Effie May Buckley, RN, MN
Choice Healing
18 Ponderosa Place
Boise, ID 83716
Phone: 208-429-8097
Website: www.choicehealing.net
Email: choicehealing@aol.com

Areas of specialty: Health Care, consultant, homeopathy, nutrition, neutriceuticals, energy medicine, diabetes, heavy metals.

ILLINOIS

Janet Fakhouri, N.D., N.C., M.S.
Custom Health, Inc.
10748 South Cook Avenue
Oak Lawn, IL. 60453
708-261-7178

James Corzine DC
Accident & Chronic Pain Center
210 West Market Street
Christopher, Illinois 62822
Phone: 618-724-9200
E-mail: jcorzine@shawneelink.net

Oscar I. Ordonez MD
Belvidere Center For Health & Nutrition
6413 Logan Avenue, Suite 104
Belvidere, Illinois 61008

Phone: (815} 544-3112
Fax: {815) 544-3114
Email: OIOMD1@netzero.com

INDIANA
Marvin Dziabis, M.D.
Health Restoration Clinic
107 W 7th St.
North Manchester, IN 46962
Phone: (260) 982-1400
Fax: (260) 982-1700
E-mail: dziabis@earthlink.net
Website: www.medical-library.net/doctors/health_restoration_clinic/

Dr. David J. Krizman
Center for Health Enrichment
322 N. Michigan St. Suite E
Plymouth, IN 46563
Phone: (574) 935-4000
Website: www.ptmc.azmyth.com

IOWA
Frank Wiewel
People Against Cancer
604 East Street – P.O. Box 10
Otho, Iowa 50569 USA
Phone: 515-972-4444
Fax: 515-972-4415
E-Mail: info@PeopleAgainstCancer.net
Website: www.PeopleagainstCancer.net

KANSAS

Bowers Natural Wellness
3450 N Rock Road Building 500 Suite 503
Wichita, KS 67226
Phone: (316) 636-5333
Fax: (316) 636-5338
E-mail: bnw@bnw.kscoxmail.com
Website: www.bowerswellness.com
Areas of specialty: Diplomate of the Chiropractic Board of Internal
Diagnosis, Certified Functional Medicine Physician.

MAINE
Sean McCloy, M.D., M.P.H.
Maine Integrative Wellness
222 Auburn St.
Portland, ME 04103
Phone: (207) 828-4299
Fax: (207) 828-5056

Email: drmccloy@mainewellness.com
Website: www.mainewellness.com

Fredric Shotz, N.D.
Maine Integrative Wellness
174 Falmouth Rd
Falmouth, Maine 04105
Phone: (207) 828-4299
Fax: (207) 828-5056

Email: drshotz@mainewellness.com
Website: www.mainewellness.com

MARYLAND

Barbara Johnson, RN
3605 Southside Avenue
Phoenix, MD 21131-173
Phone: 410-628-6877
Email: bjohnsonrn@aol.com

Sholpan Yestekov, ND
Holistic Well-being
18514 Office Park Dr.
Gaithersburg, MD 20886
Phone: 301-366-1779
Email: sholpan@nes-kz.com
Website: www.holistic-wellbeing-health.com

Areas of specialty: Alternative and complementary medicine, Poly-MVA and more to help support cancer patients.

MICHIGAN

Linda K. Hegstrand, MD, PhD
Blue Heron Academy of Healing Arts and Sciences
2040 Raybrook SE Suite 104
Grand Rapids, MI 49546
Phone: 616-974-9004
E-Mail: Lhegstrand@aol.com

Steven Margolis, M.D.
(Family Practice Physician)
Alternacare Clinic

37300 Dequindre Road, Suite 201
Sterling Heights, Michigan 48310
Phone: 586-268-0228
Fax: 586-268-7392
E-Mail:Alternacare@hotmail.com

MINNESOTA

Jean O'Hern, N.D.
Nature's Wisdom
2516 Lyndale Avenue South
Minneapolis, MN 55405
Phone: 612-872-4210
E-Mail: johern@usinternet.com

MISSISSIPPI

Dr. Arnold Smith, MD
North Central Mississippi Regional Cancer Center
1401 River Road
Greenwood, MS 38930
Phone: 662-459-7133 Fax: 662-459-7136
Website: http://www.cancernet.com/

MISSOURI

Wesley Delport, ND
Abundant Health and Wellness
4323 S. National Avenue

Springfield, MO 65810
Phone: (417) 890-7400
Toll Free: 800-528-7796
Email: abundanthealth@sbcglobal.net
Website: www.getwellnaturally.net

Stuart Hoover, NHD
Essential 2 Health
1358 E. Kingsley Street Suite C
Springfield, MO 65804
Phone: (417) 883-0115
Website: www.e2health.com

NEVADA

James W. Forsythe, M.D., H.M.D.
Medical Oncologist and Homeopath
521 Hammill Lane
Reno, Nevada 89511
Phone: (775) 827-0707
Fax: (775) 827-1006
Website: www.drforsythe.com
Email: eforsythe@sbcglobal.net

Robert Eslinger, MD
Reno Integrative Medical Center
6110 Plumas Street, Suite B
Reno, NV 89519
Phone: (775) 829-1009

Website: www.renointegrativemedicalcenter.com

Terry Pfau, MD
Renaissance Health Center
2820 W. Charleston Blvd., Suite 6
Las Vegas, NV 89102
Phone: (702) 258-7860
Website: www.terrypfau-do.md.com/

NEW JERSEY

Stuart H. Freedenfeld, MD
Stockton Family Practice
56 South Main St
Stockton, NJ 08559
Phone: 609-397-8585
E-mail: info@stocktonfp.com
Website: http://www.StocktonFP.com

Areas of Specialty: At Stockton Family Practice we have been offering cancer therapies for clients who wish complimentary support during chemotherapy or radiation treatments, for clients who have failed conventional therapies, and for those who choose not to pursue conventional chemotherapy.

We offer a wide range of services, from dietary interventions, nutritional supplements, and metabolic therapies, to acupuncture and intravenous therapies. We will develop an integrative program based on the specific needs and specific wishes of each individual.

Some of the therapies include enzymes, Antineoplastons, angiogenesis inhibitors, Vitamin C, Ozone, Poly-MVA, Haluronic acid, Ukraine and Amygdalin.

Molly Fantasia, PhD & Ronald Intelisano, DO

Associates In Preventive Medicine
1930 E. Marlton Pike, Suite J52
Cherry Hill, NJ 08003
Phone: 856-489-0505
Fax: 856-489-0435
E-mail: IVDOCS@aol.com
Website: www.cherryhillclinic.com

Areas of Specialty: Molly Fantasia, PhD – Fellow, American Association of Integrative Medicine. We provide therapy for: Auto-Immune Diseases, Cancer Support, Glutathione, Hydration Therapy, Preventative Medicine, Predictive Genomic Testing.

Allan Magaziner, DO
Magaziner Center for Wellness
1907 Greentree Road
Cherry Hill, NJ 08003
Phone: (856) 424-8222
Website: www.drmagaziner.com

NEW YORK

Richard Linchitz, MD
Jesse A. Stoff, MD
Linchitz Medical Wellness
70 Glen Street, Suite 240
Glen Cove, NY 11542
516.759.4200
Website: http://www.linchitzwellness.com
Email: info@linchitzwellness.com

Moshe Dekel
166 Elaine Drive
Oceanside, NY 11572

Phone: 516-208-6617
Fax: 516-208-6617
E-mail: doc@drdekel.com
Website: www.drdekel.com

NORTH CAROLINA

Rashid A. Buttar, DO, FACAM, FAAPM
Advanced Concepts In Alternative And Preventive Medicine
20721 Torrence Chapel Road, Suite 101 – 102
Cornelius, NC 28031
Phone: (704) 895-9355
Fax: (704) 895-9357
E-Mail: drbuttarclinic@aol.com
Website: www.drbuttar.com

Bill Crawford, M.D., Board Certified Naturopath
P.O. Box 995
Franklin, NC 28744
Phone: (828) 421-9336
Fax: (828) 349-1367

OHIO
Marcus Cobb, MD
Healthy Pursuit Medical Center
7060 Ridgetop Drive
West Chester, OH 45069
Phone: (513) 779-4325
Fax: (513) 742-1296
E-Mail: marcuslcobb@mac.com

Theodore Togliatti MD
Steven Mann DO
Insook Chung RN MSN FNP
Get Well Center
635 S. Trimble Road
Mansfield, Ohio 44906
Phone: (419) 524-2676
Fax: (419) 524-2692
E-mail: ChungGWC@aol.com

Larry Everhart, MD
Host Nutrition
3779 Attucks Drive
Powell, OH 43065
Phone: (614) 718-9800

OKLAHOMA

Mary Schrick, N.D.
Full Circle Health Clinic
3601 S. Broadway
Edmond, Oklahoma 73013
Phone: (405) 753-9355

Dr. Paul Rothwell, M.D.
Wellness and Longevity
7530 NW 23rd Street
Bethany, Oklahoma 73008
Phone: 405-787-8556
Fax: 405-787-7424
Email: info@wellnessok.com
Website: www.wellnessok.com

TEXAS

Ashok Patel, MD
500 North Highway 67
Cedar Hill, TX 75104
Phone: 972-291-4289
Email: dragpatel@yahoo.com

Dr. Exiquio Cardenas, MD, ND
Eagle Pass, TX 78852
Email: Dr.naturista@hotmail.com (available by email only)

Areas of specialty: More than 30 years without using pharmaceutical drugs. Alternative Medicine Therapeutics, Biomagnetismo, Bowen Technique, Auriculotherapy, Master Tung's Acupuncture, Reiki, Healing Touch, Vegetarianism, Herbology, Nutridetoxification, Ayurvedic...

George Allibone, MD
Houston Wellness Clinic
550 Poast Oak Blvd. Suite 330
Houston, TX 77027
Phone: (713) 808-9058
Website: www.houstonwellnessclinic.com

Jan Sims, ND
Nutritional Solutions
1213 Primrose Lane Suite 101
Denton, TX 76201
Phone: (940) 484-4391
Website: www.naturesremedydenton.com

UTAH

Jeanne Wallace, PhD, CNC
Michelle Gerencser, MS
Patrice Surley, MH, CN
Nutritional Solutions Consulting Group
1697 E. 3450 N.
N. Logan, Utah 84321
Phone: (435) 563-0053
Fax: (435) 538-8058
Email: admin@nutritional-solutions.net
Website: www.nutritional-solutions.net

VERMONT

Julian Jonas, CCH, Lic. Ac.
Center for Homeopathy of Southern Vermont
220 Western Avenue
Brattleboro, VT 05301
Office: 802-254-2928
E-mail: jjjonas@sover.net
Website: www.centerforhomeopathy.com
Areas of specialty: Constitutional homeopathy and adjunctive therapies
for acute and chronic illness.

WYOMING
Jonathan W. Singer, DO
1401 Airport Parkway, Suite 150
Cheyenne, Wyoming 82001
Phone: 307-635-4362
E-Mail: singerdo@aol.com

International Practitioners

ANTIGUA
Jose Humphreys, N.M.D., D.N.M., Ph.D
Optimum Health Clinic
P. O. Box W1280
Belvedere's Estate
St. John's, Antigua
Phone: (268) 561-2124
Fax: (268) 561-2124
Email: drjhumphreys@gmail.com

ARUBA

Carlos Viana, PhD, OMD, CAd, FACACN
Viana Natural Healing Center
Kibaima 7
Aruba, Dutch West Indies
Phone: (297) 85 1270
Fax: (297) 85 4789
E-Mail: drcarlos52@hotmail.com

AUSTRALIA

Russell Cooper, MD
60 Summerleas Rd.
Kingston, Tasmania 7050
Phone: 011-613-6239-1572

E-Mail: anubha@esat.net.au

Area of specialty: Dr. Cooper has been practicing Integrative Medicine for 18 years. He uses nutritional and environmental medicine through his practice. He uses intravenous, oral, vitamin, antioxidant, mineral, enzyme and amino acid therapies and chelation. His practice is holistic, embracing counseling and meditation for patients.

DOMINICAN REPUBLIC
George Zabrecky, M.D.
The Americas Research & Treatment Center
El Vergel #45 Ortega y Gasset
Santa Domingo, Dominican Republic
Phone: (809) 472-1238
Fax: (809) 567-8386

BAHAMAS
Dr. Sir Kevin C. King, N.D M.D.(M.A.), F.R.C.P.
The Natural Health Clinic
#4 Lucayan Plaza
Coral Road
Freeport, Bahamas
Phone: 1-242-373-8102
Fax: 1-242-373-1052
E-Mail: sir_kevinking@hotmail.com

Norman R. Gay, M.D.
Bahamas Anti-Aging Medical Institute
P.O. Box N3222
West Bay Street
Nassau, Bahamas
Phone: 1-242-328-4100
Fax: 1-242-328-4104
E-Mail: drnormangay@yahoo.com

BRITISH COLUMBIA
Jim Chan, ND
EuroMed Foundation
3331-No. 3 Road
Richmond, BC V6X 2B6
Phone: (604) 273-4372
Website: www.drjimchan.com
E-Mail: info@drjimchan.com

CYPRESS
Dr. George J Georgiou, Ph.D.,N.D.,DSc (AM).,MSc.,BSc
Holistic Medicine Practitioner DaVinci Natural Health Centre
Panayia Aimatousa 300, Aradippou 7101
Larnaca, Cyprus
Telephone: (+357) 24-82 33 22
Fax: (+357) 24- 82 33 21
E-Mail: admin@docgeorge.com
Website: www.docgeorge.com and www.collegenaturalmedicine.com

DOMINICAN REPUBLIC
George Zabrecky, M.D.
The Americas Research & Treatment Center
El Vergel #45 Ortega y Gasset
Santa Domingo, Dominican Republic
Phone: (809) 472-1238
Fax: (809) 567-8386

ITALY
Fiamma Ferraro, MD
Via Paganella 7A
00135 Roma,Italy
Phone: (+39)0635500018
Cell: (+39)3403754383
E-Mail: fer@yahoo.com
Website: www.geocities.com/fiafer

JAPAN
Andrew Wong, MD, PhD
Roppongi Dr. Andy`s Clinic of Plastic & Cosmetic
Surgery and Age Management Medicine
6/7 F Roppongi Shimada Bldg.,
4-8-7, Roppongi, Minato-ku
Tokyo, Japan 106-0032
Phone: 81-3-3401-0720
Fax: 81-3-3401-0704
E-mail: andy@drandy.com
Web Page: www.drandy.com

LEBANON
Tony Georges Lichaa, M.D.
(Specialist in Internal Medicine & Cardiology Trained at the Montreal
Heart Institute, American Board of Chelation Therapy)

Beirut Location:

The Anti-Aging and Life Rejuvenating
Medical Center
Verdun Plaza One, 2nd Floor
Beirut, Lebanon

Phone: 961 3 25 49 45
Email: tlichaa@inco.com.lb

Jounieh Location:

The Medical Center For Prevention And The Treatment Of Diseases
P.O. Box 245
Jounieh, Lebanon
Phone: 961 9 911 875
Fax: 961 9 914 195
Email: tlichaa@inco.com.lb

MANITOBA

Dr. Jim Chan, N.D.
EuroMed Foundation
3331-No. 3 Road
Richmond, BC V6X 2B6
Phone: (604) 273-4372
Email: info@drjimchan.com
Website: www.drjimchan.com

Dennis Wong, B.Sc. Pharm., FAARFM, CCN, ABAAHP
CD Whyte Ridge Pharmacy Specialty Compounding & Integrative
Consultation services
123 Scurfield Blvd.
Winnipeg, MB
Phone: 204-488-1819
Fax: 204-489-2828

CinDen Pharmacy
1600 Pembina Hwy.
Winnipeg, MB R3T 5Z2
Phone: 204-452-7989

Fax 204-452-7585
Email: dennis@cdwhyteridgerx.com
Website: www.cdwhyteridgerx.com

Area of specialty: Clinical Consultant Pharmacist /owner; Fellow, Anti-Aging, Regenerative & Functional Medicine; Certified Clinical Nutritionist; Diplomat, American Board of Anti-Aging Health Practitioners.

MEXICO
Playas de Tijuana, B.C.
Phone: 1-855-366-4673
Fax: 1-619-956-7071
Website: www.h4cmedical.com
E-mail: Info@h4cmedical.com

Recommended Therapies Could Include: Sono-Photo Dynamic Therapy, Poly MVA, Insulin Potentiation Therapy, Hyperthermia, Enzyme Therapy, IV Therapy, Iscador, Laetrile, Detoxification, and Anti-Cancer Vaccines. The anti-cancer programs at Hope4Cancer Institute are specifically designed to meet the needs of each individual patients.

Jorge Llamas, MD
Paseo Playas #400 Secc. Terrazas
Playas de Tijuana, B.C.
Mexico Phone: 664-680-1484
U.S. Phone: 619-752-9903
Cell Phone: 664-188-5533
E-mail: Dr_llamas@hotmail.com
Metabolic Therapies: Hyperthermia (Whole Body) and Local Indiba, I.P.T., Galuanotherapy, Oxygen Therapy, Homo-Acupuncture, Nutrition

Exiquio Cardenas, Medico Alapata/Naturopata

Piedras Negras, Coahuila
E-mail: Dr.naturista@hotmail.com
Areas of Specialty: Mas de 30 anos de experiencia en terapias alternativas
no farmacologicas, terapia de Bowen, biomagnetismo, auriculoterapia,
herbolaria Ayurvedica, reiki, healing touch, terapia celular, Master Tung's
acupuncture, nutricion naturista, medicina antienvejecimiento,
deintoxicacion intensiva, etc.

Clinical Trials often have specific enrollment criteria, however, one cannot select which treatment (which arm of the study) they wish participate in.

Thus, one loses control of their treatment when entering a Clinical Trial. NSABP trials are well designed and will not shirk a patient from basic established therapy; they are now to fine-tune the treatments.

A Collaborative Palliative and Oncology Care Model for Patients With Acute Myeloid Leukemia.

Detailed Description:-

The main purpose of this study is to compare two types of care - standard leukemia oncology care and standard leukemia oncology care with collaborative involvement of palliative care clinicians to see which is better for improving the experience of patients and families with AML undergoing treatment.

The investigators aim to find out whether introducing patients and families undergoing AML treatment to the palliative care team that specializes in symptom management can improve the physical and psychological symptoms that patients and families experience during their hospitalizations for their leukemia care as well as enhance the quality of patients' end of life care.

Locations:- United States, Massachusetts

Massachusetts general Hospital
Boston, Massachusetts, United States, 02114
Contact: Areej El-Jawahri, MD   617-643-4003

Principal Investigator: Areej El-Jawahri, MD

United States, North Carolina
Duke University
Durham, North Carolina, United States, 27710
Contact: Thomas LeBlanc, MD   919-684-8964
Principal Investigator: Thomas LeBlanc, MD

Principal Investigator:- Areej El-Jawahri, MD - Massachusetts General Hospital.

Tel:- 617-726-5765
Email:- ael-jawahri@partners.org

Matched Targeted Therapy For High-Risk Leukemias.

Detailed Description:-

This study will determine whether it is possible to use profiling results and determine a matched targeted therapy for patients with leukemia. It will describe the range of mutations found in patients with leukemia with this type of profiling, and describe the clinical outcomes of patients who receive a matched targeted therapy.

Our tissues and organs are made up of cells. Cancer occurs when the molecules that normally control cell growth are damaged. The damage results in unchecked cell growth which causes a tumor, a collection of cancer cells. The damage is referred to as an alteration.

There are different types of cancer-causing alterations. Genes are the part of cells that contain the instructions which tell our cells how to make the right proteins to grow and work. Genes are composed of DNA letters that spell out these instructions.

By participating in this study, the participant's leukemia cells will be tested for cancer causing alterations. This testing is called leukemia profiling. The leukemia profiling will be performed using bone marrow or blood that has already been obtained during a clinical test. Alternately, the profiling may be done on leukemia cells that are planned to be obtained as part of routine clinical care.

Contacts and Locations:-
Locations:- United States, California

UCSF Helen Diller Family Comprehensive Cancer Center
San Francisco, California, United States, 94158
Contact: Mignon Loh, MD   415-514-0853   Lohm@peds.ucsf.edu
Principal Investigator: Mignon Loh, MD

United States, Colorado
Children's Hospital Colorado
Aurora, Colorado, United States, 80045
Contact: Kelly Maloney, MD 720-777-6740
Kelly.Maloney@ucdenver.edu
Principal Investigator: Kelly Maloney, MD

United States, Maryland
Johns Hopkins Hospital
Baltimore, Maryland, United States, 21287
Contact: Patrick Brown, MD   410-955-8817
Pbrown2@jhmi.edu
Principal Investigator: Patrick Brown, MD

United States, Massachusetts
Dana Farber Cancer Institute
Boston, Massachusetts, United States, 02215
Contact: Yana Pikman, MD
617-632-4754
YPIKMAN@PARTNERS.ORG
Principal Investigator: Yana Pikman, MD
Sub-Investigator: Lewis B Silverman, MD
Sub-Investigator: Andrew Place, MD, PhD

United States, New York
Columbia University Medical Center
New York, New York, United States, 10032
Contact: Maria-Luisa Sulis, MD
212-305-5808
Mls95@cumc.columbia.edu
Principal Investigator: Maria-Luisa Sulis, MD

United States, Pennsylvania
Children's Hospital of Philadelphia
Philadelphia, Pennsylvania, United States, 19404
Contact: Sarah Tasian, MD
267-425-0118
TasianS@email.chop.edu
Principal Investigator: Sarah Tasian, MD
United States, Washington

Seattle Children's Hospital
Seattle, Washington, United States, 98105
Contact: Todd Cooper, MD
206-987-1533
Todd.Cooper@seattlechildrens.org
Principal Investigator: Todd Cooper, MD

Contacts:-
Contact: Yana Pikman, MD
617-632-4754
YPIKMAN@PARTNERS.ORG

Contact: Andrew Place, MD, PhD
617-632-2313
andrew_place@dfci.harvard.edu

Evaluation of Adverse Long-term Effects in Young Adult Survivors of Acute Leukemia (LEA-JA).

Purpose:- Taking into account the specificities of adolescent and young adult cancer patients led agencies (in particular the French National Cancer Institute INCa, through the last Cancer Plan), to initiate projects targeting this population. Acute leukemia is among the most common cancers in adolescents and young adults. Recent therapeutic advances now allow hope for a cure in about 50% of this population.

The issue of post-cancer is therefore of particular importance for young adults with cancer. Our aim is to establish the health determinants in young adult leukemia survivors and to compare the frequency of these effects and their explanatory factors to the data collected in children or adolescent leukemia survivors program (LEA). 90 patients followed up at the Institut Paoli-Calmettes cancer center and Nice University Hospital have been identified and would be included in this study.

Collected data will include information on the initial disease and its treatments, physical sequelae (fertility, thyroid function, heart function, visual function, secondary tumors, viral infections, lung function, bone metabolism, iron metabolism, metabolic syndrome, osteonecrosis, alopecia), quality of life, social and occupational integration and relationship with care system.

Copyright - 2017. Published by Cancer Group Institute. www.cancergroup.com 124

Locations:- France
Institut Paoli-Calmettes
Marseille, France, 13009
Contact: Dominique Genre, MD
0033491223778
drci.up@ipc.unicancer.fr
Principal Investigator: Norbert VEY, MD PhD

Contacts:-
Contact: Dominique GENRE, MD
0033491223778
drci.up@ipc.unicancer.fr

Contact: Jihane Pakradouni, PharmD PhD
0033491223778
drci.up@ipc.unicancer.fr

Multi-center Prospective Cohort of Childhood Leukemia: Determinants of Health and Quality of Life of the Patients After Treatment for an Acute Leukemia During Childhood or Adolescence - LEA.

Purpose:-

Regular advances in cancer treatment have dramatically improved the prognosis of children and adolescents with acute leukemia (AL), raising with a great acuity the problem of the late physical side effects, social integration, quality of life of the patients and their family as well as identification of the determinants of these outcomes.
Large nationwide and international cohorts developed in general population (I4C, EPIC ELF...) are restricted to the study of childhood

cancers occurrence. In addition, the national registries (French, European) of childhood cancers are designed to evaluate incidence and mortality, but not to produce individual detailed data on the follow-up and outcome of these children. Answering these questions supposes a comprehensive multidisciplinary approach resting on prospective cohorts of cancer survivors, specifically exploring the outcome of these children.

These cohorts allow to identify prognostic factors of the health condition and social integration, and to propose adapted strategies of follow-up. The Childhood Cancer Survivor Study (CCSS), which remains the most important study, only concerns the North-American populations and rests on a self-reported follow-up assessment. In France, the LEA study, initiated in 2004 could answer some of these questions, but the representativeness and the size of the population (study initially limited to two areas PACA-Corsica and Lorraine) remain insufficient to study uncommon events. Similar approaches are conducted in Europe through the broad collaborative Pancare network, to which the LEA program is associated.

Locations:- France
Assistance Publique Hopitaux de Marseille
Marseille, France, 13354
Contact: PASCAL AUQUIER
pascal.auquier@ap-hm.fr

Evaluation of Splenic Irradiation in Chronic Lymphatic Leukemia.

Purpose:-

Retrospective evaluation on the effect of splenic irradiation on clinical and hematological response and toxicity in patients with chronic lymphatic leukemia (CLL).

Locations:- Netherlands

Maastro Clinic
Maastricht, Netherlands
Contact: Jacques Borger, Dr.

Principal Investigator:- Jacques Borger, Dr.
Email:- jacques.borger@maastro.nl
Sub-Investigator:- Roel Schlijper

CAR-T Therapy for Central Nervous System B-cell Acute Lymphocytic Leukemia.

Purpose:- This study will evaluates the safety and efficacy of Chimeric antigen receptor T cells (CAR-T) in treating central nervous system B-cell acute lymphocytic leukemia.

Locations:- China
The First Affiliated Hospital of Soochow University
Suzhou, China
Contact: Depei Wu, Ph.D
Tel:- 86-13328008851
Email:- slxue@suda.edu.cn

Lei Yu, Ph.D
Tel:- 86-13818629089
Email:- ylyh188@163.com

Burkitt Leukemia - Dose-Adjusted Etoposide, Prednisone, Vincristine, Cyclophosphamide, and Ofatumumab (EPOCH - O).

Purpose:- The goal of this clinical research study is to learn if adding ofatumumab/rituximab to the standard combination of DA-EPOCH (dose-adjusted etoposide, prednisone, vincristine, and cyclophosphamide) can help control the disease in patients with newly diagnosed or relapsed/refractory Burkitt leukemia or relapsed/refractory ALL. The safety of this drug combination will also be studied.

Locations:- United States, Texas
University of Texas MD Anderson Cancer Center
Houston, Texas, United States, 77030

Contact:- Elias Jabbour, MD
Tel:- 713-792-4764
E-mail:- ejabbour@mdanderson.org

N-PhenoGENICS: Neurocognitive-Phenome, Genome, Epigenome and Nutriome In Childhood Leukemia Survivors (N-PhenoGENICS).

Purpose:- To find possible therapeutic targets to help prevent long-term brain and behavioural side effects in survivors of childhood leukemia that may have been caused by chemotherapy (Treatment-Related late Adverse Neuro-Cognitive Effects: TRANCE). The study hypothesis is that genetic variations of the elements in the folate-related cycles and methotrexate disposition networks are associated with the TRANCE phenotype of childhood.

Locations:- Canada, Ontario
The Hospital for Sick Children
Toronto, Ontario, Canada
Contact:- Laura Hopf
Tel:- 416-813-8285
Email:- laura.hopf@sickkids.ca

Contact:- Patrick Te
Tel:- 416-813-7654 ext 201828
Email:- patrick.te@sickkids.ca

Principal Investigator:- Dr. Shinya Ito
E-mail:- shinya.ito@sickkids.ca
Tel:- 416-813-5776

Samples From Leukemia Patients and Their Donors to Identify Specific Antigens.

Purpose:- The purpose of this project is to develop a process to identify highly personalized antigens that are uniquely expressed by the patient's own leukemia cells that can be used for cellular immune therapy.

Locations:- United States, California

University of California San Diego
La Jolla, California, United States, 92093
Contact:- Jesika Reiner, MPH
Tel:- 858-822-5364
Email:- JReiner@ucsd.edu

Lenalidomide in Acute Leukemias and Chronic Lymphocytic Leukemia.

Purpose:- Lenalidomide has properties of thalidomide and appears to have some activity against cancer in laboratory tests. Researchers are still learning how lenalidomide works against cancer in patients. Some ways that this drug seems to produce anti-cancer effects include through stimulating the immune system and blocking blood vessels contributing to cancer growth. The current study will explore different dose levels in patients to gather more information about lenalidomide.

Purpose:- This study will assess the maximum tolerated dose of lenalidomide in patients with relapsed or refractory acute leukemias and chronic lymphocytic leukemias. Toxicity or side effects within patients will also be evaluated. Other purposes of this study include analyzing preliminary clinical activity, pharmacokinetics, and pharmacodynamics. Pharmacokinetics refers to the activity of drugs in the body over a period of time, including how drugs are absorbed, distributed, localized in tissues, and excreted. Pharmacodynamics refers to the bodily processes that lead the drug to effect cancer and other cellular components in the body.

Treatment:- Study participants will be given lenalidomide through intravenous infusions once every 28 days. A 28-day period constitutes a cycle. Since this study will assess the maximum tolerated dose of lenalidomide, some study participants will receive different amounts of this drug compared to others depending upon when each individual enrolls in the study. Each group of 3 to 6 study participants will receive a higher dose of lenalidomide until the maximum tolerated dose is established.

Several tests will be performed throughout the study, including bone marrow biopsies. Imaging exams will be conducted as well. Treatments will be discontinued due to disease growth or intolerable adverse effects. Lenalidomide administration will be repeated for 12 or more cycles in patients that experience clinical benefit.

Locations:- United States, Ohio

Ohio State University Medical Center

A354 Starling-Loving Hall
320 W 10th Ave
Columbus, OH 43210

Principal Investigator:- Leslie Andritsos, MD
Tel:- 614-366-3802
Email:- leslie.andritsos@osumc.edu

Phase I Dose Escalation of BAY1143572 in Subjects With Acute Leukemia.

Purpose:- To determine the safety, tolerability, pharmacokinetics, maximum tolerated dose, and recommended Phase II dose of BAY1143572 in a once-daily or an intermittent dosing schedule in subjects with advanced acute leukemia.

Official Title:- An Open-label Phase I Dose-escalation Study to Characterize the Safety, Tolerability, Pharmacokinetics, and Maximum Tolerated Dose of BAY1143572 Given in a Once-daily or an Intermittent Dosing Schedule in Subjects With Advanced Acute Leukemia.

Locations:- United States, Massachusetts
Dana-Farber Cancer Institute
Boston, Massachusetts, United States, 02215

United States, New Jersey
Hackensack University Medical Center
Hackensack, New Jersey, United States, 07601

United States, New York
Columbia University Medical Center
New York, New York, United States, 10032

Copyright - 2017. Published by Cancer Group Institute. www.cancergroup.com 131

United States, South Carolina
Medical University of South Carolina
Charleston, South Carolina, United States, 29425

United States, Tennessee
Vanderbilt University Medical Center
Nashville, Tennessee, United States, 37232

Germany
Universitätsklinikum der Johann Wolfgang Goethe Universität
Frankfurt, Hessen, Germany, 60596

Universitätsklinikum Münster (UKM)
Münster, Nordrhein-Westfalen, Germany, 48149

Medizinische Fakultät Carl Gustav Carus
Dresden, Sachsen, Germany, 01307

Therapy Optimisation for the Treatment of Hairy Cell Leukemia.

Purpose:- The trial will test the effectiveness and toxicity of subcutaneous treatment with one cycle of cladribine in patients with hairy cell leukemia requiring treatment.

They have to be untreated so far or may be pretreated with alpha-interferon.

Primary Outcome Measures:- Determination of the rate of complete remissions after one cycle with subcutaneous cladribine.

Copyright - 2017. Published by Cancer Group Institute. www.cancergroup.com 132

Secondary Outcome Measures:- Rate of complete remissions in patient who still have detectable residual disease. A second cycle of cladribine after an interval of 4 months following the first cycle.

Justus-Liebig-University
University Hospital
Medicinal Clinic IV
Germany

Principal Investigator:- Mathias J Rummel, Prof. Dr.
Email:- mathias.rummel@innere.med.uni-giessen.de
Tel:- +4964198542, Ext: 650

Contact:- Juergen Barth
Tel:- +4964198542 ext 603
Email:- juergen.barth@innere.med.uni-giessen.de

Sorafenib for Prophylaxis of Leukemia Relapse in Allo-HSCT Recipients With FLT3-ITD Positive AML.

Purpose:- The purpose of this study is to evaluate the efficacy of sorafenib for prophylaxis of leukemia relapse in allogeneic stem cell transplant (Allo-HSCT) recipients with FLT3-ITD positive acute myeloid leukemia (AML).

Detailed Description:- Internal tandem duplication of FMS-like tyrosine kinase 3 (FLT3-ITD) mutations have been reported in 20%-30% of patients with acute myeloid leukemia (AML). FLT3-ITD-positive AML patients have an inferior survival, primarily due to lower complete remission (CR) rate and higher relapse rate. Although allogeneic hematopoietic stem cell transplantation (allo-HSCT) improves the outcomes of some FLT3-ITD-positive AML, a significant number will suffer disease recurrence after allo-HSCT.

Sorafenib, an inhibitor of multiple kinases including FLT3, has shown promising activity in FLT3-ITD-positive AML. Recent studies have shown that sorafenib monotherapy or in combination with chemotherapy are effective in attaining CR, but they do not have significant improvement in relapse. Currently, prophylactic use of sorafenib after allo-HSCT has been rarely reported, and whether it can improve outcomes of FLT3-ITD-positive AML remains unclear.

Locations:- China, Guangdong
Department of Hematology
Nanfang Hospital
Southern Medical University
Guangzhou
Guangdong
China, 510515

Contact:- Li Xuan
Tel:- +86-020-61641613
Email:- 356135708@qq.com

First Report:- Five Years' Experience of the Acute Leukemia Work Group (PR-GTLA).

Purpose:- The purpose of this study is to describe the incidence, clinic characteristics, biological and survival in Lymphoblastic Leukemia patients in Mexico City reference hospitals.

Locations:- Mexico

Instituto Nacional de Ciencias Médicas y Nutrición Salvador Zubirán
Mexico Distrito Federal
Mexico 1400
Contact:- Roberta Demichelis, Doctor
Tel:- 015554870900 ext 2700
Email:- robertademichelis@gmail.com

Contact:- Karla Espinoza, Doctor
Tel:- 015556280400 ext 60035

C-X-C Chemokine Receptor 4 in Chronic Lymphocytic Leukemia.

Purpose:- Chronic lymphocytic leukemia is the most common type of chronic leukemia, accounting for approximately 40% of all leukemias and mainly affecting older individuals. As it has a highly variable clinical course, identification of molecular and biological prognostic markers has provided new insights into the risk stratification of patients with chronic lymphocytic leukemia.

Detailed Description:- Prognosis depends primarily on the stage of the disease at diagnosis. There is a correlation between disease stage and median survival. However, about 50% of patients in early stage will develop more advanced disease. Also there is marked variation in disease progression amongst patients with similar Stages.

Extreme clinical heterogeneity is one of the hallmark features of chronic lymphocytic leukemia despite the identification of genetic and phenotypic markers that correlate with prognosis, the biological basis of this clinical variability remains unclear.

In addition, the interactions of chronic lymphocytic leukemia cells with the microenvironment in secondary lymphoid tissues and the bone

Copyright - 2017. Published by Cancer Group Institute. www.cancergroup.com

marrow are known to promote chronic lymphocytic leukemia cell survival and proliferation.

The median age at diagnosis is 72 years, in the last decades chronic lymphocytic leukemia is more often diagnosed also in younger individuals, with almost 15% Of patients Of 55 years old or younger. There is a gender predisposition, As men are more frequently affected by chronic lymphocytic leukemia than women (male: female ratio of 1.5-2:1).

C-X-C chemokine receptor type 4 (CXCR4) is a chemokine and chemokine receptor pair playing critical roles in tumorigenesis. Overexpression of C-X-C chemokine receptor type 4 is a hallmark of many hematological malignancies including acute myeloid leukemia, chronic lymphocytic leukemia and non-Hodgkin's lymphoma, and generally correlates with a poor prognosis. A highly potent competitive antagonist of C-X-C chemokine receptor type 4 recently has been identified with suppression of cancer cells aggressiveness in a variety of cancers.

The protein-coupled receptor C-X-C chemokine receptor type 4 is activated by stromal cell-derived factor 1 and is involved in the control of migration and homing of cells notably for engraftment of normal and neoplastic hematopoietic cells in the bone marrow (BM).

Bruton's tyrosine kinase (BTK) is a key player in B-cell antigen receptor (BCR) signaling that regulates B-cell growth. In addition to B-cell antigen receptor signaling, Bruton's tyrosine kinase participates in signal transduction through growth-factor receptors, Toll-like receptors, integrins and G-protein-coupled receptors such as C-X-C chemokine receptor type 4 and C-X-C chemokine receptor type 5. Bruton's tyrosine kinase inhibition results in impaired C-X-C chemokine receptor type 4 chemokine receptor surface expression, signaling and function in chronic lymphocytic leukemia.

Copyright - 2017. Published by Cancer Group Institute. www.cancergroup.com 136

inhibition of Bruton's tyrosine kinase function would lead to a loss of tumor volume by preventing replenishment after spontaneous or drug-induced death, and by subverting leukemia cell retention in and homing back to sustaining tissue niches. Decrease C-X-C chemokine receptor type 4 delays disease progression and prolongs survival.

Locations:- United States - Ohio
The University of Toledo
2801 W. Bancroft
Toledo
OH - 43606-3390

Contact:- Eman Mohamed Salah, MD
Tel:- 015556280400 ext 60035
Health Science Campus
Ruppert Health Center
Room # 0012

Phone: 419.383.3685
Email:- Emansalah.eldin@yahoo.com
Tel:- 01028030966

Acute Lymphoblastic Leukemia Therapies Informed by Genomic Analyses.

Purpose:- Previous work performed by University of New Mexico Comprehensive Cancer Center (UNMCCC) investigators has revealed previously unknown genomic mutations in children, adolescents, and young adults with high-risk B and T cell precursor acute lymphoblastic leukemia (ALL). Using genomic and next generation DNA sequencing technologies, these investigators revealed that 14% of children with high-risk ALL have "Philadelphia chromosome-like" ("Ph-like") ALL. Patients with this form of ALL were found to have a significantly increased risk of treatment failure and death.

Further work revealed that there are more than 40 distinct gene rearrangements and fusions that can result in Ph-like ALL. Cell lines and human leukemic cells expressing some of these different gene fusions were sensitive to currently available drugs. This suggests that Ph-like ALL patients with these specific distinct gene fusions should be targeted in future clinical trials to be treated with appropriate therapy. Further work is also needed to identify other potentially targetable genetic alterations in ALL patients.

Therefore, the goal of this study is to perform genomic screening of all newly diagnosed ALL patients seen at UNM and to use this information to enroll patients onto available National Clinical Trial Network (NCTN) clinical trials. If an appropriate NCTN trial is not available, best clinical management will be pursued.

Primary Outcome Measures:- ALL characterization: Low Density Array. Newly diagnosed ALL patients at UNMCCC will undergo Low Density Array (LDA) card screening (a gene expression classifier for Ph-like ALL) at initial diagnosis. The proportion of LDA status (positive vs. negative) and its 95% confidence interval will be calculated based on the exact binomial distribution.

ALL characterization: Next Generation Sequencing. Newly diagnosed ALL patients at UNMCCC will undergo Next Generation Sequencing (NGS) at initial diagnosis. NGS (exomic and transcriptomic) of a sufficient read depth (500-700x) will be employed to detect clonal heterogeneity at diagnosis. Statistical analysis will be primarily descriptive (e.g. frequency (proportion) of various mutations will be calculated).

ALL characterization: SNP analysis. Newly diagnosed ALL patients at UNMCCC will undergo Molecular Determination of Genetic Ancestry (using a panel of single nucleotide polymorphisms (SNPs)) at initial diagnosis. Statistical analysis will be primarily descriptive (e.g. frequency (proportion) of SNPs and genetic ancestry groups will be calculated).

Detailed Description:- The work performed by UNMCCC investigators and others as described briefly above has provided major insights into the biologic and clinical features and the genomic landscape of Ph-like ALL, which is strikingly heterogeneous.

Gene expression profiling and RNA/transcriptomic, exome, and whole genome sequencing have identified several distinct subclasses of kinase activating lesions in 91% of the Ph-like ALL cases studied to date, most commonly kinase and cytokine receptor gene rearrangements and fusions. UNMCCC investigators are now collaborating with Children's Oncology Group (COG) and the adult National Cancer Institute (NCI) Cooperative Groups (Southwest Oncology Group (SWOG), Eastern Cooperative Oncology Group (ECOG) - American College of Radiology Imaging Network (ACRIN), The Alliance) to develop national clinical trials for pediatric, adolescent and young adult (AYA), and adult ALL patients that incorporate their genomic diagnostic screens, molecular diagnostics, and next generation sequencing studies to identify underlying genomic lesions in ALL and target patients to appropriate therapeutic regimens.

In this feasibility study, next generation sequencing (NGS) technologies will inform an acute lymphoblastic leukemia risk classification system, which may be adapted to identify patients who might benefit from targeted therapies; such patients will be targeted to NCTN National Treatment trials or UNMCCC-sponsored trials where appropriate, through detailed genomic data analysis performed under College of American Pathologists (CAP)/CLIA conditions and in individual case discussions in a Molecular Tumor Board.

In addition, the association of race and ethnicity with the spectrum of ALL-associated genomic mutations in the New Mexico and regional ALL population, which includes a significant proportion of underrepresented minorities, will be studied. This may ultimately allow for the development of an ancestry-based risk classification system.

Locations:- United States, New Mexico
University of New Mexico Comprehensive Cancer Center
Albuquerque, New Mexico, United States, 87131

Contact: Valerie Parks, RN
Tel:- 505-925-0390
Email:- vparks@salud.unm.edu

Principal Investigator:- Jodi Mayfield, MD
Tel:- 505-272-4461
Email:- jrmayfield@salud.unm.edu

Phase I Trial of Cabozantinib in Patients With Relapsed or Refractory Acute Myeloid Leukemia.

Purpose:- This clinical trial is evaluating a drug called **cabozantinib** as a possible treatment for acute myeloid leukemia (AML). This research study is a Phase I clinical trial. Phase I trials test the safety of an investigational drug or combination of drugs. Phase I studies also try to define the appropriate dose of the investigational drug to use for further studies. This means that the FDA has not approved giving cabozantinib for use in patients, including patients with your type of cancer.

The study drug cabozantinib works by inhibiting several different proteins which are believed to be involved in the growth and multiplication of the cancerous cells associated with acute myeloid

Copyright - 2017. Published by Cancer Group Institute. www.cancergroup.com | 140 leukemia. This drug has been used in other research studies and information from those other research studies suggests that this drug may help to prevent cancer growth.

The primary purpose of this research study is to determine the highest dose of Cabozantinib that can safely be given without severe or unmanageable side effects. The dose identified in this study will be used in future research studies that seek to determine the role of cabozantinib as a treatment for AML.

Primary Outcome Measures:- Maximum tolerated dose (MTD) of cabozantinib in patients with advanced acute myeloid leukemia. To define the maximum tolerated dose (MTD) of cabozantinib in patients with advanced acute myeloid leukemia.

Locations:- United States, Massachusetts
Beth Israel Deaconess Medical Center
Boston, Massachusetts, United States, 02215

Massachusetts General Hospital
Zero Emerson Place, Suite 118
Boston, Massachusetts, United States, 02215

Principal Investigator:- Amir Fathi, MD
Tel:- 617-724-1124
Email:- afathi@mgh.harvard.edu

Collecting and Storing Blood, Bone Marrow, and Other Samples From Patients With Acute Leukemia, Chronic Leukemia, or Myelodysplastic Syndromes.

Purpose:- As one of the nation's largest cooperative cancer treatment groups, the Alliance for Clinical Trials in Oncology (Alliance) is in a unique position to organize a Leukemia Tissue Bank. The member institutions diagnose hundreds of patients with leukemia or myelodysplastic syndrome each year, and uniformly treat these patients with chemotherapy regimens. The Alliance offers centralized data management for the clinical history, the classification of the leukemia and myelodysplastic syndrome, cytogenetics, flow cytometric analysis, treatment and follow-up.

The highly skilled health care providers at each member institution are familiar with obtaining informed consent, completing data questionnaires and shipping specimens. There currently exists a central processing facility where samples are prepared for a variety of cellular and molecular studies. Hence, the patient resources, the health care providers, and a processing facility for a Leukemia Tissue Bank are all in place. What is needed, however, and is addressed in the current protocol, is a formal mechanism to procure bone marrow, blood and normal tissue from patients with hematologic malignancies who are to be enrolled on Alliance (Cancer and Leukemia Group B [CALGB]) treatment studies.

Locations:- United States, California
Camino Medical Group - Treatment Center

Mountain View, California, United States, 94040
Pismo Beach, California, United States, 93449
Naval Medical Center - San Diego
San Diego, California, United States, 92134

UCSF Helen Diller Family Comprehensive Cancer Center
San Francisco, California, United States, 94115

United States, Connecticut
Helen and Harry Gray Cancer Center at Hartford Hospital
Hartford, Connecticut, United States, 06102-5037

United States, Delaware
Tunnell Cancer Center at Beebe Medical Center

Copyright - 2017. Published by Cancer Group Institute. www.cancergroup.com 142

Lewes, Delaware, United States, 19958

CCOP - Christiana Care Health Services
Newark, Delaware, United States, 19713

United States, District of Columbia
Lombardi Comprehensive Cancer Center at Georgetown University Medical Center
Washington, District of Columbia, United States, 20007

Washington Cancer Institute at Washington Hospital Center
Washington, District of Columbia, United States, 20010

United States, Florida
Michael and Dianne Bienes Comprehensive Cancer Center at Holy Cross Hospital
Fort Lauderdale, Florida, United States, 33308

Ella Milbank Foshay Cancer Center at Jupiter Medical Center
Jupiter, Florida, United States, 33458

CCOP - Mount Sinai Medical Center
Miami Beach, Florida, United States, 33140

Florida Hospital Cancer Institute at Florida Hospital Orlando
Orlando, Florida, United States, 32803-1273

United States, Illinois
Illinois CancerCare - Bloomington
Bloomington, Illinois, United States, 61701

St. Joseph Medical Center
Bloomington, Illinois, United States, 61701

Illinois CancerCare - Canton
Canton, Illinois, United States, 61520

University of Illinois Cancer Center
Chicago, Illinois, United States, 60612-7243

Veterans Affairs Medical Center - Chicago Westside Hospital
Chicago, Illinois, United States, 60612

University of Chicago Cancer Research Center
Chicago, Illinois, United States, 60637-1470

Eureka Community Hospital
Eureka, Illinois, United States, 61530

Illinois CancerCare - Eureka
Eureka, Illinois, United States, 61530

Evanston Hospital
Evanston, Illinois, United States, 60201-1781

Galesburg Clinic, PC
Galesburg, Illinois, United States, 61401

Illinois CancerCare - Macomb
Macomb, Illinois, United States, 61455

BroMenn Regional Medical Center
Normal, Illinois, United States, 61761

Community Cancer Center
Normal, Illinois, United States, 61761

Illinois CancerCare - Community Cancer Center
Normal, Illinois, United States, 61761

Community Hospital of Ottawa
Ottawa, Illinois, United States, 61350

Oncology Hematology Associates of Central Illinois, PC - Ottawa
Ottawa, Illinois, United States, 61350

Cancer Treatment Center at Pekin Hospital
Pekin, Illinois, United States, 61554

Illinois CancerCare - Pekin
Pekin, Illinois, United States, 61603

Proctor Hospital
Peoria, Illinois, United States, 61614

CCOP - Illinois Oncology Research Association
Peoria, Illinois, United States, 61615

Oncology Hematology Associates of Central Illinois, PC - Peoria
Peoria, Illinois, United States, 61615

Methodist Medical Center of Illinois
Peoria, Illinois, United States, 61636

OSF St. Francis Medical Center
Peoria, Illinois, United States, 61637

Illinois CancerCare - Peru
Peru, Illinois, United States, 61354

Illinois Valley Community Hospital
Peru, Illinois, United States, 61354

Illinois CancerCare - Spring Valley
Spring Valley, Illinois, United States, 61362

United States, Indiana
Elkhart Clinic, LLC

Elkhart, Indiana, United States, 46514-2098

Michiana Hematology-Oncology, PC - Elkhart
Elkhart, Indiana, United States, 46514

Elkhart General Hospital
Elkhart, Indiana, United States, 46515

Howard Community Hospital
Kokomo, Indiana, United States, 46904

Center for Cancer Therapy
LaPorte Hospital and Health Services
La Porte, Indiana, United States, 46350

Suniti Medical Corporation
Merrillville, Indiana, United States, 46410

Michiana Hematology-Oncology, PC - South Bend
Mishawaka, Indiana, United States, 46545-1470

Saint Joseph Regional Medical Center
Mishawaka, Indiana, United States, 46545-1470

Michiana Hematology Oncology PC - Plymouth
Plymouth, Indiana, United States, 46563

CCOP - Northern Indiana CR Consortium
South Bend, Indiana, United States, 46601

Memorial Hospital of South Bend
South Bend, Indiana, United States, 46601

Michiana Hematology Oncology PC - La Porte
Westville, Indiana, United States, 46391

United States, Iowa
Hematology Oncology Associates of the Quad Cities
Bettendorf, Iowa, United States, 52722

Iowa Blood and Cancer Care
Cedar Rapids, Iowa, United States, 52402

Holden Comprehensive Cancer Center at University of Iowa
Iowa City, Iowa, United States, 52242-1002

Veterans Affairs Medical Center - Iowa City
Iowa City, Iowa, United States, 52246

United States, Kansas
Menorah Medical Center
Overland Park, Kansas, United States, 66209

Saint Luke's Hospital - South
Overland Park, Kansas, United States, 66213

CCOP - Kansas City
Prairie Village, Kansas, United States, 66208

United States, Maine
Harold Alfond Center for Cancer Care
Augusta, Maine, United States, 04330

CancerCare of Maine at Eastern Maine Medical Center
Bangor, Maine, United States, 04401

United States, Maryland
Greenebaum Cancer Center at University of Maryland Medical Center

Baltimore, Maryland, United States, 21201

National Naval Medical Center

Bethesda, Maryland, United States, 20889-5600

Union Hospital of Cecil County
Elkton MD, Maryland, United States, 21921

United States, Massachusetts
Massachusetts General Hospital
Boston, Massachusetts, United States, 02114

Dana-Farber/Brigham and Women's Cancer Center
Boston, Massachusetts, United States, 02115

Dana-Farber/Harvard Cancer Center at Dana-Farber Cancer Institute

Boston, Massachusetts, United States, 02115

Addison Gilbert Hospital
Gloucester, Massachusetts, United States, 01930

United States, Michigan
Lakeland Regional Cancer Care Center - St. Joseph
Saint Joseph, Michigan, United States, 49085

Lakeside Cancer Specialists, PLLC
Saint Joseph, Michigan, United States, 49085

United States, Minnesota
St. Luke's Hospital Cancer Care Center
Duluth, Minnesota, United States, 55805

Veterans Affairs Medical Center - Minneapolis
Minneapolis, Minnesota, United States, 55417

Masonic Cancer Center at University of Minnesota
Minneapolis, Minnesota, United States, 55455

United States, Missouri
Southeast Cancer Center
Cape Girardeau, Missouri, United States, 63703

Ellis Fischel Cancer Center at University of Missouri - Columbia
Columbia, Missouri, United States, 65203

Goldschmidt Cancer Center
Jefferson City, Missouri, United States, 65109

Saint Luke's Cancer Institute at Saint Luke's Hospital
Kansas City, Missouri, United States, 64111

North Kansas City Hospital
Kansas City, Missouri, United States, 64116

Heartland Hematology Oncology Associates, Incorporated
Kansas City, Missouri, United States, 64118

Research Medical Center
Kansas City, Missouri, United States, 64132

Saint Luke's East - Lee's Summit
Lee's Summit, Missouri, United States, 64086

Saint Joseph Oncology, Incorporated
Saint Joseph, Missouri, United States, 64507

Siteman Cancer Center at Barnes-Jewish Hospital - Saint Louis
Saint Louis, Missouri, United States, 63110

Missouri Baptist Cancer Center
Saint Louis, Missouri, United States, 63131

United States, Nebraska
Saint Francis Cancer Treatment Center at Saint Francis Memorial Health

Center
Grand Island, Nebraska, United States, 68803

Callahan Cancer Center at Great Plains Regional Medical Center
North Platte, Nebraska, United States, 69103

UNMC Eppley Cancer Center at the University of Nebraska Medical Center

Omaha, Nebraska, United States, 68198-6805

United States, Nevada
University Medical Center of Southern Nevada
Las Vegas, Nevada, United States, 89102

CCOP - Nevada Cancer Research Foundation
Las Vegas, Nevada, United States, 89106

Sunrise Hospital and Medical Center
Las Vegas, Nevada, United States, 89109

United States, New Hampshire
New Hampshire Oncology - Hematology, PA at Payson Center for Cancer
Care
Concord, New Hampshire, United States, 03301

New Hampshire Oncology - Hematology, PA - Hooksett
Hooksett, New Hampshire, United States, 03106

Lakes Region General Hospital
Laconia, New Hampshire, United States, 03246

Norris Cotton Cancer Center at Dartmouth-Hitchcock Medical Center
Lebanon, New Hampshire, United States, 03756-0002

Norris Cotton Cancer Center at Catholic Medical Center
Manchester, New Hampshire, United States, 03102

United States, New Jersey
Cancer Institute of New Jersey at Cooper - Voorhees
Voorhees, New Jersey, United States, 08043

United States, New York
Roswell Park Cancer Institute
Buffalo, New York, United States, 14263-0001

CCOP - Hematology-Oncology Associates of Central New York
East Syracuse, New York, United States, 13057

Charles R. Wood Cancer Center at Glens Falls Hospital
Glens Falls, New York, United States, 12801

Queens Cancer Center of Queens Hospital
Jamaica, New York, United States, 11432

Monter Cancer Center of the North Shore-LIJ Health System
Lake Success, New York, United States, 11042

CCOP - North Shore University Hospital
Manhasset, New York, United States, 11030

Don Monti Comprehensive Cancer Center at North Shore University
Hospital
Manhasset, New York, United States, 11030

Long Island Jewish Medical Center
New Hyde Park, New York, United States, 11040

New York Weill Cornell Cancer Center at Cornell University
New York, New York, United States, 10021

Mount Sinai Medical Center
New York, New York, United States, 10029

SUNY Upstate Medical University Hospital
Syracuse, New York, United States, 13210

Veterans Affairs Medical Center - Syracuse
Syracuse, New York, United States, 13210

United States, North Carolina
Mission Hospitals - Memorial Campus
Asheville, North Carolina, United States, 28801

Lineberger Comprehensive Cancer Center at University of North Carolina
- Chapel Hill
Chapel Hill, North Carolina, United States, 27599-7295

Blumenthal Cancer Center at Carolinas Medical Center
Charlotte, North Carolina, United States, 28232-2861

Presbyterian Cancer Center at Presbyterian Hospital
Charlotte, North Carolina, United States, 28233-3549

Batte Cancer Center at Northeast Medical Center
Concord, North Carolina, United States, 28025

Duke Cancer Institute
Durham, North Carolina, United States, 27710
Wayne Memorial Hospital, Incorporated
Goldsboro, North Carolina, United States, 27534

Leo W. Jenkins Cancer Center at ECU Medical School
Greenville, North Carolina, United States, 27834

Pardee Memorial Hospital
Hendersonville, North Carolina, United States, 28791

Kinston Medical Specialists

Kinston, North Carolina, United States, 28501

Cleveland Regional Medical Center
Shelby, North Carolina, United States, 28150

Iredell Memorial Hospital
Statesville, North Carolina, United States, 28677

Forsyth Regional Cancer Center at Forsyth Medical Center
Winston-Salem, North Carolina, United States, 27103

Wake Forest University Comprehensive Cancer Center
Winston-Salem, North Carolina, United States, 27157-1096

United States, Ohio
Arthur G. James Cancer Hospital and Richard J. Solove Research Institute
Ohio State University
Comprehensive Cancer Center
Columbus, Ohio, United States, 43210-1240

United States, Oklahoma
Cancer Care Associates - Norman
Norman, Oklahoma, United States, 73071

Oklahoma University Cancer Institute
Oklahoma City, Oklahoma, United States, 73104

Cancer Care Associates - Mercy Campus
Oklahoma City, Oklahoma, United States, 73120

United States, Pennsylvania
Western Pennsylvania Cancer Institute at Western Pennsylvania Hospital

Pittsburgh, Pennsylvania, United States, 15224-1791

Copyright - 2017. Published by Cancer Group Institute. www.cancergroup.com

United States, Rhode Island
Rhode Island Hospital Comprehensive Cancer Center
Providence, Rhode Island, United States, 02903

Miriam Hospital
Providence, Rhode Island, United States, 02906

United States, South Carolina
McLeod Regional Medical Center
Florence, South Carolina, United States, 29501

Cancer Centers of the Carolinas - Faris Road
Greenville, South Carolina, United States, 29605

Cancer Centers of the Carolinas - Grove Commons
Greenville, South Carolina, United States, 29605

Greenville Hospital Cancer Center
Greenville, South Carolina, United States, 29605

Cancer Centers of the Carolinas - Eastside
Greenville, South Carolina, United States, 29615

CCOP - Greenville
Greenville, South Carolina, United States, 29615

Cancer Centers of the Carolinas - Greer Medical Oncology
Greer, South Carolina, United States, 29650

Cancer Centers of the Carolinas - Seneca
Seneca, South Carolina, United States, 29672

Cancer Centers of the Carolinas - Spartanburg
Spartanburg, South Carolina, United States, 29307

United States, Vermont

Copyright - 2017. Published by Cancer Group Institute. www.cancergroup.com 154

Mountainview Medical
Berlin, Vermont, United States, 05602

Fletcher Allen Health Care - University Health Center Campus
Burlington, Vermont, United States, 05401

United States, Virginia
Danville Regional Medical Center
Danville, Virginia, United States, 24541

Ravenel Oncology Center at Memorial Hospital of Martinsville and Henry
County
Martinsville, Virginia, United States, 24115

Virginia Commonwealth University Massey Cancer Center
Richmond, Virginia, United States, 23298-0037

Principal Investigator:- Michael Caligiuri, MD
Tel:- 614-292-2220
Email:- michael.caligiuri@osumc.edu

Ohio State University Comprehensive Cancer Center
The Ohio State University College of Medicine
370 W. 9th Ave.
Columbus, OH 43210

Prospective Study on the Feasibility of Plasma FLT3-Ligand Assay to Achieve a First Estimate of Its Prognostic Value on the Outcome of Patients Treated Intensively for Acute Leukemia (FLAM/FLAL).

Purpose:- Despite advances in their classification and treatment, acute leukemia remain incurable disease for the majority of patients. It is necessary to identify new prognostic markers of survival and new therapeutic targets to improve prognosis. Some studies have shown that Fms-like tyrosine kinase 3-ligand (FLT3-L) could be interesting from this. A more recent study from our group testing a novel therapy in acute lymphoblastic leukemia, showed an increase of this marker in the blood of patients responding to treatment.

The aim of our prospective, non-interventional study is to measure the plasma levels of FLT3-L at different times of the management of patients with acute lymphoblastic leukemia but also myeloid. For this, analyzes of the samples collected in the usual care will be conducted to study the relationship between the plasma concentration of FLT3-L and outcomes. If there is any link, the FLT3-L could serve as a predictor of treatment response.

Locations:- France
Nantes University Hospital
immeuble Deurbroucq
5 allée de l'île Gloriette
44093 Nantes Cedex 1
Nantes, France, 44093

Principal Investigator:- Pierre Peterlin, Dr
Tel:- 02 40 08 74 18
Email:- pierre.peterlin@chu-nantes.fr

Contact:- Patrice CHEVALLIER, Pr
Tel:- 02 40 08 39 94
Email:- patrice.chevallier@chu-nantes.fr

BI 836858 Dose Escalation in Patients With Refractory or Relapsed Acute Myeloid Leukemia and in Patients in Complete Remission With High Risk to Relapse.

Purpose:- Patients with acute myeloid leukemia who experience a relapse after at least one prior regimen may be enrolled in this trial. In addition, acute myeloid leukemia patients who are in complete remission with high risk to relapse may be eligible for this trial. The trial will examine whether monotherapy with BI 836858 is safe and tolerable at escalating dose levels.

Locations:- United States, Connecticut
Yale University School of Medicine
New Haven, Connecticut, United States, 06510

United States, Illinois
Robert H. Lurie - Comprehensive Cancer Center, Chicago
Chicago, Illinois, United States, 60611

United States, Ohio
Ohio State University
Columbus, Ohio, United States, 43210

Principal Investigator:- Boehringer Ingelheim Call Center
Tel:- 1-800-243-0127
Email:- clintriage.rdg@boehringer-ingelheim.com

ChEmo-Genomics Based Treatment of Acute Myeloid Leukemia (CeGAL).

Purpose:- Adult acute myeloid leukemia (AML) is a heterogeneous hematologic malignancy associated with poor prognosis, especially after relapse. High-throughput genomic studies have highlighted the importance of molecular alteration in the pathophysiology, clinical evolution and treatment response of AML. In addition, identification of specific gene mutation can be targeted by specific inhibitors, opening the way to personalized treatments. However, only a limited number of gene mutations are druggable or actionable, highlighting the need for additional information to guide treatment choices. Among them, new Drug Screening Tests (DST) allow for the screening of library of hundreds of drugs to ex-vivo patient-derived AML cells.

A combination of genomic and pharmacologic approaches might therefore improve prediction of drug effects. There is an urgent need to bring these approaches into the clinic but feasibility trials are necessary before incorporating them into treatments strategies.The proposed study is a prospective multicentre feasibility study of a combined "chemo-genomic" approach in patients with advanced AML.

Locations:- France

Institut Paoli-Calmettes, Département Enseignement et Formation,
232 Boulevard Sainte-Marguerite
BP 156 - 13273 Marseille - Cedex 9
Marseille, France

Contact: Dominique GENRE, MD
Email:- drci.up@ipc.unicancer.fr

Contact:- Jihane PAKRADOUNI, PharmD,PhD
Tel:- (33)4 91 22 37 78
Email:- drci.up@ipc.unicancer.fr

Principal Investigator:- Norbert VEY, MD
Email:- veyn@marseille.fnclcc.fr

Biomarkers in Blood and Bone Marrow Samples From Patients With Acute Lymphoblastic Leukemia.

Purpose:- **RATIONALE:-** Studying samples of blood and bone marrow from patients with cancer in the laboratory may help doctors learn more about changes that occur in DNA and identify biomarkers related to cancer.

PURPOSE:- This research study is studying biomarkers in blood and bone marrow samples from patients with acute lymphoblastic leukemia.

To perform high-resolution, genome-wide profiling of DNA copy number alterations and loss-of-heterozygosity in samples from adult patients with acute lymphoblastic leukemia (ALL) obtained at diagnosis.

To perform candidate gene resequencing of diagnostic ALL samples.

To examine correlation of genetic alterations with outcome.

To examine the correlation between microarray multi-gene and multi-exon expression signatures with specific alterations and outcome.

To understand genetic events that contribute to the formation, development, and relapse of adult ALL by integrating the copy number and sequence alterations with the multi-gene signatures, and by comparing these data with data already generated in pediatric ALL.

Locations:- United States, Tennessee
St. Jude Children's Research Hospital
262 Danny Thomas Place
Memphis, TN 38105-3678

Principal Investigator:- James Downing, MD
Email:- james.downing@stjude.org
Tel:- Phone: 901-595-3956

LY2510924, Idarubicin and Cytarabine in Patients With Relapsed or Refractory Acute Myeloid Leukemia.

Purpose:- The goal of this clinical research study is to learn about the safety of LY2510924 in combination with cytarabine and idarubicin in patients with relapsed or refractory AML. We will also study if

Copyright - 2017. Published by Cancer Group Institute. www.cancergroup.com

LY2510924 in combination with cytarabine and idarubicin can help to control relapsed or refractory AML.

LY2510924 is designed to help cancer cells move from the bone marrow into the bloodstream, where they are exposed to chemotherapy (in this case, cytarabine and idarubicin).

Locations:- United States, Texas
University of Texas MD Anderson Cancer Center
Houston, Texas, United States, 77030

Principal Investigator:- Marina Konopleva, MD, PHD
Email:- mkonople@mdanderson.org
Tel:- 713-794-1628

Combination Chemotherapy in Treating Young Patients With Newly Diagnosed Acute Lymphoblastic Leukemia.

Purpose:- RATIONALE: Drugs used in chemotherapy work in different ways to stop the growth of cancer cells, either by killing the cells or by stopping them from dividing. Giving more than one drug (combination chemotherapy) may kill more cancer cells.

PURPOSE:- This phase II trial is studying how well combination chemotherapy works in treating young patients with newly diagnosed acute lymphoblastic.

Locations:- United States, Illinois
University of Chicago
5841 S Maryland Ave
Chicago, IL 60637

Principal Investigator:- Wendy Stock, M.D.
E-mail:- wstock@medicine.bsd.uchicago.edu

Treatment of Relapsed and/or Chemotherapy Refractory CD33 Positive Acute Myeloid Leukemia by CART-33 (CART33).

Purpose:- RATIONALE: Placing a tumor antigen chimeric receptor that has been created in the laboratory into patient autologous or donor-derived T cells may make the body build immune response to kill cancer cells.

PURPOSE:-This clinical trial is to study genetically engineered lymphocyte therapy in treating patients with CD33 positive acute myeloid leukemias that is relapsed (after stem cell transplantation or intensive chemotherapy) or refractory to further chemotherapy.

PRIMARY OBJECTIVES:-
1. Determine the safety and feasibility of the chimeric antigen receptor T cells transduced with the anti-CD33 vector (referred to as CART-33 cells).

2. Determine duration of in vivo survival of CART-33 cells. RT-PCR (reverse transcription polymerase chain reaction) analysis of whole blood will be used to detect and quantify survival of CART-33 TCR zeta:CD137 and TCR (T-cell receptor) zeta cells over time.

Locations:- China, Beijing
Biotherapeutic Department and Pediatrics
Department of Chinese PLA General Hospital
Hematological Department
Affiliated Hospital of Changzhi Medical College
Beijing, Beijing, China, 100853

Principal Investigator:- Weidong Han, Dr.
Tel:- 86-10-13651392893
Email:- hanwdrsw@sina.com

Contact:- Xuliang Shen, Dr.
Tel:- 86-355-13015365546
Email:- shenxlcyp@sohu.com

Trial of Immune Reconstitution With Activated T-Cells Following Lymphodepleting Chemotherapy in Patients With Chronic Lymphocytic Leukemia (CLL).

Purpose:- Patient's immune systems are often damaged by chemotherapy or by CLL. Researchers want to learn if giving T-cells (immune cells) that have been expanded and specially processed in the laboratory (activated) will help CLL patients' immune systems recover after chemotherapy. This may help lower the chance of infections.

The goal of this clinical research study is to learn if an activated T-cell infusion, when given with or without lenalidomide, can help to restore patients' immune systems when given after chemotherapy (rituximab and fludarabine with cyclophosphamide or bendamustine). The safety of this treatment combination will also be studied.

Researchers also want to learn if the activated T-cells may also be able to kill cancer cells.

Primary Outcome Measures:- Success of Autologous T Cells for Immune Restoration in Participants with Chronic Lymphocytic Leukemia (CLL).

Success defined as achievement of a target activated T-cell dose of 1×10^8 +/- 20% and lack of dose limiting toxicity (DLT). DLT defined as any grade 4 or higher non-hematologic toxicity or grade 3 or 4 allergy/immunology toxicity, allergic reaction or urticaria grade 3 or higher (CTC v4.03 CTCAE) by +90 days after T cell infusion, grade 2 or greater autoimmune phenomena or grade 4 or higher hematologic toxicity (with the exception of any preexisting AE due to prior treatment or due to disease) deemed related to T cells and occurring by day +90 after T cell infusion.

Feasibility of Autologous T Cells for Immune Restoration in Participants with Chronic Lymphocytic Leukemia (CLL) [Time Frame: 90 days after T-cell infusion].

Feasibility defined as achievement of the target T cell dose (1 x 108 +/- 20%) in > 50% of patients enrolled.

Locations:- United States, Texas
University of Texas
MD Anderson Cancer Center
Houston, Texas, United States, 77030

Principal Investigator:- Chitra M. Hosing, MD
Tel:- 713-794-5745
Email:- cmhosing@mdanderson.org

A Phase 1b Study Evaluating the Safety and Tolerability of ABT-199 in Combination With Rituximab in Subjects With Relapsed Chronic Lymphocytic Leukemia and Small Lymphocytic Lymphoma.

Purpose:- This is a Phase 1b, open-label, multicenter study evaluating the safety and tolerability of ABT-199 in combination with rituximab in up to 50 subjects with Relapsed Chronic Lymphocytic Leukemia and Small Lymphocytic Lymphoma. The primary objectives of this study are to assess the safety profile, to determine the maximum tolerated dose and establish the Recommended Phase Two Dose of ABT-199 when administered in combination with rituximab.

The dose escalation portion of the study will include approximately 30 subjects. Once the recommended phase two dose and schedule have been determined, up to 20 additional subjects will be enrolled in an expanded safety portion of the study. Subjects who meet criteria for CR, CRi, or

MRD-negative PR during the study may discontinue ABT 199. If disease progression occurs, as defined by iwCLL NCI/WG criteria for tumor response, subjects may re-initiate ABT-199.

Primary Outcome Measures:- Assess the safety profile, to determine the maximum tolerated dose and Recommended Phase Two Dose of ABT-199 when administered in combination with rituximab (R) in subjects with relapsed chronic lymphocytic leukemia and small lymphocytic lymphoma. [Time Frame: Continuous dosing at designated dose level up to Month 6. At end of combination treatment, ABT-199 monotherapy may continue up to 4 years following the date of the last subject enrolled. If disease progression occurs, subjects may re-initiate ABT-199].

Protocol-defined events, which are attributed as having a reasonable possibility of being related to the administration of ABT-199 and/or rituximab, or cannot be attributed by the investigator to a clearly identifiable cause such as tumor progression, concurrent illness, underlying disease or concomitant medication, will be considered a dose limiting toxicity.

Locations:- United States, California
UCSD Moores Cancer Center, US /ID# 70398
La Jolla, California, United States, 92093

United States, Illinois
Northwestern University /ID# 71593
Chicago, Illinois, United States, 60611

United States, New York
North Shore University Hospital /ID# 71813
New Hyde Park, New York, United States, 11042

United States, North Carolina
Duke Cancer Center /ID# 71393
Durham, North Carolina, United States, 27710

Australia
Peter MacCallum Cancer Centre /ID# 70394
East Melbourne, Australia, 3002

Royal Melbourne Hospital /ID# 70393
Parkville, Melbourne, Australia, 3050

Principal Investigator:- Su Y Kim, MD

MEK Inhibitor 162 Relapsed and/or Refractory Acute Myeloid Leukemia (AML) and Poor Prognosis, Not Suitable for or Unwilling to Receive Standard Therapy.

Purpose:- The goal of Phase 1 of this clinical research study is to find the highest tolerable dose of MEK162 that can be given to patients with advanced leukemia.

The goal of Phase 2 of this clinical research study is to learn if MEK162 can help to control AML in older patients with advanced leukemia. The safety of this drug will also be studied.

Primary Outcome Measures:- Maximum Tolerated Dose (MTD) of MEK 162 in Participants with Advanced Leukemias [Time Frame: 28 days]. Maximum tolerated dose is the highest dose level in which <2 patients of 6 develop dose limiting toxicity (DLT).

Locations:- United States, Texas
University of Texas MD Anderson Cancer Center
Houston, Texas, United States, 77030

Principal Investigator:- Farhad Ravandi-Kashani, MD
Tel:- 713-745-0394
Email:- fravandi@mdanderson.org

Copyright - 2017. Published by Cancer Group Institute. www.cancergroup.com 165

B-type Chronic Lymphocytic Leukemia (B-CLL) Subgroups: Maturation Stage and Gene Expression.

Purpose:- B type chronic lymphocytic leukemia (B-CLL) is the most prevalent leukemia in the western world. It is a disease that occurs primarily in aging individuals and occurs more frequently in males than females. Although B-CLL was considered a homogeneous condition, recent studies by our laboratory and others suggest that B-CLL cases can be divided into two subgroups.

These sub-groups can be identified by either the presence or the absence of mutations in antibody genes and/or by the percentage of B-CLL cells expressing a particular protein called CD38. These two sub-groups (unmutated antibody genes high percent CD38 and mutated antibody genes low percentage CD38) follow strikingly clinically different courses. For example, the unmutated/CD38+ group experiences a much more aggressive disease and these patients almost invariably die much sooner than the cases in the other group.

In addition, the patients in the mutated CD38+ group require much more chemotherapy than mutatedlCD38-. Finally, surprisingly there is a much higher representation of males in the poor outcome unmutated CD38 group than in the better outcome group. The reasons for these differences in clinical outcome and gender bias are unknown.

Locations:- United States, New York
Feinstein Institute for Medical Research
Manhasset, New York, United States, 11030

Principal Investigator:- Yasmine Kieso, MSCR
Tel:- 516-562-3467
Email:- ykieso@nshs.edu

Study of the Combination of Low-Intensity Chemotherapy and Ponatinib in Patients With Philadelphia Chromosome (Ph)-Positive and/or BCR-ABL Positive Acute Lymphoblastic Leukemia (ALL).

Purpose:- The goal of this clinical research study is to learn how well ponatinib combined with low-intensity chemotherapy may control Philadelphia chromosome-positive (Ph+) or BCR-ABL positive acute lymphoblastic leukemia (ALL) in patients who are at least 60 years old.

In elderly patients with ALL, intensive chemotherapy is effective but causes a lot of side effects, some of which are very serious and can be life-threatening. Researchers want to learn if using low-intensity chemotherapy in this study can achieve the same effect as high-intensity chemotherapy in the long run but with fewer side effects.

Ph+ and BCR-ABL positive are types of genetic mutations (changes).

The safety and effectiveness of the study drug combined with low-intensity chemotherapy will also be studied.

Primary Outcome Measures:- Complete Molecular Response (CMR) in Newly Diagnosed Ph-Positive and/or BCR-ABL-Positive Participants [Time Frame: 12 weeks].

CMR defined as normalization of the peripheral blood and bone marrow with 5% or less blasts in normocellular or hypercellular marrow with a granulocyte count of 1 x 109/L or above, and platelet count of 100 x 109/L. Complete resolution of all sites of extramedullary disease is required for CR.

Overall Response (OR)in Relapsed/Refractory Acute Lymphoblastic Leukemia [Time Frame: 8 weeks].

Overall response defined as complete response (CR) + complete response with hematologic improvement (CRi) in participants with relapsed/refractory disease.

Copyright - 2017. Published by Cancer Group Institute. www.cancergroup.com 167

Locations:- United States, Texas
University of Texas MD Anderson Cancer Center
Houston, Texas, United States, 77030

Principal Investigator:- Hagop Kantarjian, MD
Tel:- 713-792-7026
Email:- hkantarjian@mdanderson.org

Autologous ROR1R-CAR-T Cells for Chronic Lymphocytic Leukemia (CLL).

Purpose:- Gene transfer is a process in which the DNA (genetic material) of certain cells is changed. In this study, gene transfer will be performed on a type of white blood cell (called T cells) to recognize leukemia cells in the same person the T cells were collected from.

The goal of this clinical research study is to learn if it is safe to give these genetically-changed T cells back to patients with CLL/SLL. Researchers also want to learn if these cells can help to attack CLL/SLL cells.

Locations:- United States, Texas
University of Texas MD Anderson Cancer Center
Houston, Texas, United States, 77030

Principal Investigator:- William G. Wierda, MD, PHD, BS
Tel:- 713-745-0428
Email:- wwierda@mdanderson.org

Vitro Study of Tigecycline to Treat Chronic Myeloid Leukemia.

Purpose:- Chronic myeloid leukemia (CML) is a myeloproliferative neoplasm companies with the BCR-ABL fusion gene encoded by the

Philadelphia (Ph) chromosome. The BCR-ABL fusion protein (the formation of the chimeric gene BCR/ABL on chromosome 22 and a reciprocal ABL/BCR on chromosome 9,it has no expanded name) plays key role on CML leukemogenesis by activating its downstream signaling pathway of survival and proliferation.

Imatinib, a targeted competitive inhibitor of a BCR-ABL tyrosine kinase, changed the clinical treatment and prognosis of CML. As its optimized generation, other tyrosine kinase inhibitors (TKIs), dasatinib and nilotinib have more potent anti-leukemic activity and less side-effect. However, acquired resistance to TKIs is one of the main obstacles to effective CML treatment and is involved in gene amplication of ABL tyrosine kinase point mutations.

The outcomes of patients with these ABL tyrosine kinase point mutations have linked to worse prognosis and higher mortality generally. Metabolic adaptations are common in cancer cells, and cancer cells become more dependent on mitochondrial biogenesis.

Tigecycline, as a broad-spectrum antibiotics, inhibits mitochondrial biogenesis as it's an interesting "side-effect".In recent study,researchers indicated that tigecycline can eradicate cancer stem cells by targeting mitochondrial. Here, the investigators test tigecycline's anti-leukemic activity to chronic myeloid leukemia in vitro.

Detailed Description:- In this study, the investigators collected bone marrow(BM) or/and peripheral blood(PB) mononuclear cells from patients with chronic myeloid leukemia.Patients could be in different stages of chronic myeloid leukemia pre-treatment.Additionally, the investigators also selected some healthy volunteers as comparison.

Firstly, the investigators analyzed mitochondrial biogenesis and basal metabolic characteristic of mononuclear cells from patients and healthy volunteers.

Secondly, the investigators tested the cell viability and apoptosis after tigecycline treatment.Thirdly,the investigators detected the changes of cell mitochondrial biogenesis and metabolic characteristic in the same study sample after tigecycline stimulation. Finally,the investigators analyzed the correlation between sensitivities of mononuclear cells to tigecycline and patients' clinical parameters and survival outcome.

Locations:- China, Guangdong
Department of Hematology
Nanfang Hospital
Guangzhou
Guangdong, China, 510515

Principal Investigator:- Xiaoli Liu, MD
Tel:- 86-020-61641616
Email:- lxl2405@126.com

Contact:- Na Xu, MD
Tel:- 86-020-61641615
Email:- 292347668@qq.com

Dose Escalation Trial of WT1-Sensitized T Cells for Residual or Relapsed Leukemia After Allogeneic Hematopoietic Progenitor Cell Transplantation.

Purpose:- This study will test the safety of giving you specialized white cells from your donor. They are called WT1 sensitized T cells. They have been grown in the lab and are immunized against a protein.

The protein is called the Wilms' tumor protein, or WT1. Your leukemic cells make too much of this protein. We want to learn whether the WT1 sensitized T cells will attack the protein and kill the leukemia cells.

Primary Outcome Measures:- Assess toxicity of in vitro expanded allogeneic WT1 peptide-specific T-cells derived from transplant donor, when given to patients with leukemia or other WT1+ hematologic malignancy having relapsed after transplant or persistent minimal residual disease, [Time Frame: conclusion of the study].

Locations:- United States, New York
Memorial Sloan Kettering Cancer Center
New York, New York, United States, 10065

Principal Investigator:- Susan Prockop, MD
Tel:- 212-639-6715
Email:- prockops@mskcc.org

Multidrug Resistance Genes in Patients With Acute Myeloid Leukemia.

Purpose:- This research trial studies multidrug resistance genes in patients with acute myeloid leukemia. Studying samples of bone marrow or blood from patients with cancer in the laboratory may help doctors learn more about changes that may occur in deoxyribonucleic acid (DNA) and identify biomarkers related to cancer. It may also help doctors learn more about drug resistance and how patients respond to treatment.

Primary Outcome Measures:- Correlation of common single nucleotide polymorphisms (SNPs) and haplotypes of the 3 multidrug resistance genes (P-glycoprotein [Pgp], multidrug resistance-associated protein (MRP-1) and breast cancer resistance protein [BCRP]) with treatment outcome. Effect of ATP-binding cassette (ABC) B1, ABCC1, and ABCG2 polymorphisms on treatment outcome.

Locations:- United States, Indiana
Fort Wayne Medical Oncology and Hematology
Fort Wayne, Indiana, United States, 46845

Principal Investigator:- Maria R. Baer, MD

Tel:- 410-328-8708
Email:- mbaer@umm.edu

A Clinical Research of CAR T Cells Targeting CD19 Positive Malignant B-cell Derived Leukemia and Lymphoma.

Purpose:- The main purpose of this research is to verify the safety of CD19 targeted chimeric antigen receptor T cells and to determine the proper dosage of CAR T cells infused.

Primary Outcome Measures:- Adverse events of each patient. Determine the toxicity profile of the CD19 targeted CAR T cells with Common Toxicity Criteria for Adverse Effects (CTCAE).

Locations:- China, Chongqing
Southwest Hospital of Third Millitary Medical University
Chongqing, Chongqing, China, 400000

Principal Investigator:- Cheng Qian, MD, PhD
Tel:- 008615086883400 or 0086-023-68765461
Email:- cqian3184@163.com

Contact:- Zhi Yang, PhD
Tel:- 0086-13206140093
Email:- Lystch@qq.com

Axitinib and Bosutinib for Patients With Chronic Myeloid Leukemia in Chronic, Accelerated or Blastic Phases.

Objectives:- Primary:

Chronic Phase Cohort:- To assess the rate of major cytogenetic response

(MCyR) of an alternating schedule of axitinib and bosutinib in patients with chronic myeloid leukemia, chronic phase (CML-CP) after failure of/intolerance to >/= 3 tyrosine kinase inhibitors (TKIs) using standard response criteria.

Advanced Phase Cohort: - Phase I Portion: To determine the recommended phase II doses (RPTDs) of axitinib and bosutinib in combination in patients with CML in accelerated phase (CML-AP) or blast phase (CML-BP). (AP patients must have received >1 prior TKI).

Advanced Phase Cohort: - Phase II Portion: To evaluate the rate of major hematologic response (MaHR) of combined treatment with axitinib and bosutinib in patients with CML-AP or CML-BP using standard response criteria. (AP patients must have received >1 prior TKI).

Locations:- United States, Texas
University of Texas MD Anderson Cancer Center
Houston, Texas, United States, 77030

Principal Investigator:- Prithviraj Bose, MD
Tel:- 713-792-7747
Email:- pbose@mdanderson.org

Alternative Splicing and Leukemia Initiating Cells (ASLIC).

Purpose:- Aberrant RNA splicing and mutations in spliceosome complex in acute myeloid leukemia (AML) are frequent. It have been shown that some splicing variants had a prognostic value in AML.

AML are characterized by their propensity to relapse because of the persistence of leukemia initiating cells (LICs).

The aim of this study is to determine the splice variants on AML initiator cells and define a splicing pattern.

Primary Outcome Measures:- Polymerase chain reaction.

Transcriptome analysis to determine the splicing variants on acute myeloid leukemia initiator cells.

The analysis will focus on the gene encoding ABCA3 transporter and genes known to be mutated in patients with acute myeloid leukemia (FLT3, NPM1, c-Kit, N et K-RAS).

The duration of selection of samples is estimated to be one month.

Ribonucleic acid sequencing [Time Frame: 1 month]

Transcriptome analysis to determine the splicing variants on acute myeloid leukemia initiator cells.

The analysis will focus on the gene encoding ABCA3 transporter and genes known to be mutated in patients with acute myeloid leukemia (FLT3, NPM1, c-Kit, N et K-RAS).

The duration of selection of samples is estimated to be one month.

Locations:- France
Service d'hématologie du Centre Hospitalier Lyon Sud
Pierre-Bénite, France, 69310

Principal Investigator:- Etienne PAUBELLE, MD, PhD
Tel:- 04 78 86 22 50 ext +33
Email:- Etienne.paubelle@chu-lyon.fr

Contact:- Erice WATTEL, MD, PhD
b 04 78 86 22 60 ext +33
Email:- eric.wattel@chu-lyon.fr

Proteasome Inhibition in Acute Promyelocytic Leukemia.

Purpose:- The clinical outcome of relapsed acute promyelocytic leukemia (APL) is poor with current standard of care approaches. Additionally, standard of care warrants an autologous stem cell transplant to be done once molecular remission is achieved. Unfortunately, the majority of our patients cannot afford this procedure. We have previously reported the clinical outcome of relapsed patients who were managed without a stem cell transplants and showed that the event free survival at 5 years is less than 35%.

Pre-clinical data reported from our laboratory demonstrates that there is significant synergy between arsenic trioxide (ATO; which is the accepted standard of care agent for relapsed APL) and Bortezomib (a proteasome inhibitor). We have evaluated this combination extensively in-vitro and this data was accepted as an oral presentation at the American Society of Hematology (ASH) meeting in 2011. More recently we have also reported the potential mechanism for this synergy (Poster at ASH 2012).

We also have mouse model data which supports these findings. We plan to move this combination of ATO based therapy combined with Bortezomib to a Phase II clinical trial to validate these observations. The anticipated potential is that we will have a combination therapy that is less expensive, cost effective and safe with comparable clinical outcomes to those treated with the more expensive standard of care which includes an autologous stem cell transplant and which the majority of our patients cannot afford.

Locations:- India
Department of Haematology
Christian Medical College
Vellore, TN, India, 632004

Principal Investigator:- Vikram Mathews
Tel:- +91 416 228 2500

Copyright - 2017. Published by Cancer Group Institute. www.cancergroup.com 175

Email:- vikram@cmcvellore.ac.in

Daratumumab in Subjects with Relapsed/Refractory Acute Myelogenous Leukemia or High-Risk Myelodysplastic Syndrome.

Purpose:- The goal of this clinical research study is to learn if daratumumab can help to control acute myelogenous leukemia (AML) or high-risk myelodysplastic syndrome (MDS) that is refractory (does not respond to treatment) or relapsed (comes back after being treated).

The safety of this drug will also be studied.

Primary Outcome Measures:- Overall Response (OR) of Daratumumab in Subjects With Relapsed/Refractory Acute Myelogenous Leukemia or High-Risk Myelodysplastic Syndrome [Time Frame: 12 weeks].

Overall response (OR), defined as achievement of complete remission (CR), CR with incomplete platelet recovery (CRp), partial remission (PR), morphologic leukemia-free state or marrow CR.

Locations:- United States, Texas
University of Texas MD Anderson Cancer Center
Houston, Texas, United States, 77030

Principal Investigator:- Gautam Borthakur, MBBS - M.D.
Tel:- 713-563-1586
Email:- gborthak@mdanderson.org

Predictive Clinical and Biological Parameters in Acute Leukemia, Myelodysplastic Syndromes and Myeloproliferative Disorders- HEMATO-BIO-IPC-2013-015 (HEMATO-BIO).

Purpose:- HEMATO-BIO-IPC-2013-015 is a monocenter prospective longitudinal study. Our aim is to define predictive clinical and biological factors in acute leukemia, myelodysplastic syndromes and myeloproliferative disorders by using genomics, genetics and epigenetics, in vitro and in vivo drug sensitivity studies, and translational immunology and immunomonitoring studies.

HEMATO-BIO primary outcome measure is to identify molecular, genomic and epigenetic, pharmacologic and immunophenotypic alteration in acute leukemia, myelodysplastic syndromes and myeloproliferative disorders by collecting, at diagnosis and/or complete remission and/or relapse:

• tumor samples: marrow aspiration, blood sampling.

• non-tumor samples: skin biopsy, buccal swab from 300 patients treated at our cancer center.

Locations:- France
Institut Paoli-Calmettes
Marseille, France, 13009

Principal Investigator:- Norbert VEY, MD,PhD
Tel:- 33 (0) 491223695
Email:- veyn@marseille.fnclcc.fr

Role of Microparticles in the Coagulopathy of Acute Promyelocytic Leukemia.

Purpose:- Although the clinical application of differentiation therapy has made great success in the treatment of acute promyelocytic leukemia (APL), early fatal bleeding remains an unsolved problem which accounts for the main reason of induction failure in APL patients. The clinical manifestation of both serious bleeding and thrombosis illustrate the complexity of the pathogenesis of coagulopathy in APL.

Despite extensive research, the pathogenesis of coagulopathy in APL is still unclear. Microparticles, 0.11µm in diameter, are small membrane vesicles released to circulation by blood cells and vascular endothelial cells during activation or apoptosis. Microparticles (MPs) derived from different cells types all exert procoagulant activity mediated by phosphatidylserine (PS) and carry some basic substances derived from their origin cells. Also, the biological activity of microparticles is often significantly higher than that of the cells they come from.

According to these problems and background knowledge, our project aims to observe the roles of microparticles derived from APL cells and the procoagulant or profibrinolytic activating factors resided on these microparticles in the pathogenesis of coagulopathy in APL, and the effects of different induction therapies, chemotherapeutic drugs or differentiation agents on these microparticles and their procoagulant or profibrinolytic activating factors.

To carry out this study, microparticles are obtained from patients who undergo different induction therapies at different time points or from primary bone marrow APL cells which are treated by different drugs in vitro at different time points, the expressions and activities of five procoagulant or profibrinolytic activating factors, which are highly expressed in APL cells, PS exposure and the functional state of these microparticles, will be dynamically monitored.

Further study of the pathogenesis of coagulopathy in APL can provide clues and help for deep understanding of clinical manifestations, guiding clinical treatment as well as judging prognosis, and establishing theoretical basis for exploring new treatment.

Primary Outcome Measures:- Change From Baseline in the Levels and Cellular Origin of MPs at 5 Weeks [Time Frame: 5 weeks].

• Demonstration that the some procoagulant or profibrinolytic activating factors expressed on MP in APL patients' plasma associate with the thrombin generating capacity and fibrinolytic activity of patients' plasma.

Locations:- China, Heilongjiang
The First Affiliated Hospital of Harbin Medical University
Harbin, Heilongjiang, China, 150001

Principal Investigator:- Jin Zhou, MD, PhD
Tel:- 008645185555951
Email:- zhoujin1111@126.com

Monitoring and Treatment of Relapsed Leukemia Following Allogeneic Hematopoietic Stem Cell Transplantation in Children.

Purpose:- This study aims to monitor patients for relapse of the leukemia following allogeneic Hematopoietic Stem Cell Transplantation (HSCT) in order to identify patients early in relapse, with a low burden of disease, when interventions may be more successful by monitoring of peripheral blood lineage specific chimerism. Once disease has been confirmed, patients will initiate a novel combination of bortezomib and pravastatin.

Locations:- United States, District of Columbia
Children's National Medical Center
Washington, District of Columbia
United States, 20010

Principal Investigator:- Reuven Schore, MD
Tel:- 202-476-2800
b rschore@childrenational.org

Contact:- Maggie Holly
Tel:- 202-476-5532
Email:- mholly@childrensnational.org

ONC201 in Relapsed/Refractory Acute Leukemias and High-Risk Myelodysplastic Syndromes (HR-MDS).

Purpose:- The goal of Phase I of this clinical research study is to find the highest tolerable dose of ONC201 that can be given to patients with relapsed or refractory AML, ALL, or MDS.

The goal of Phase II of this study is to learn if the dose of ONC201 found in Phase I can help to control the disease. The safety of the study drug will be studied in both phases of this study. This is the first study using ONC201 in humans. ONC201 is in a very early stage of development for use in humans. Providing direct medical benefit to you is not the purpose of this study.

While Phase II will look at the effectiveness of the study drug, the main purpose of this study is to learn about the safety of the drug.

Primary Outcome Measures:-

- Maximum Tolerated Dose (MTD) of ONOC201 in Relapsed or Refractory Acute Myelogenous Leukemia (AML), Myelodysplastic Syndrome (MDS) or Acute Lymphoblastic Leukemia (ALL) [Time Frame: 21 days]

  MTD is defined as the highest dose level in which 6 patients have been treated with at most 1 instance of dose limiting toxicity (DLT). Toxicities defined according to Common Terminology Criteria for Adverse Events (CTCAE) version 4.0. DLT defined as a clinically significant adverse event or abnormal laboratory value assessed as unrelated to disease progression, intercurrent illness, or concomitant medications and occurring during the first cycle on study that meets any of the following criteria:

    o CTCAE grade 3 AST (SGOT) or ALT (SGPT) for > 7 days

    o CTCAE grade 4 AST (SGOT) or ALT (SGPT) of any duration

- o   All other clinically significant NCI common terminology criteria that are CTCAE grade 3 or 4 (except for electrolyte disturbances responsive to correction within 24 h, diarrhea, nausea and vomiting that responds to standard medical care).

Locations:- United States, Texas

University of Texas MD Anderson Cancer Center

Houston, Texas

United States, 77030

Principal Investigator:- Gautam Borthakur, MBBS

Tel:- 713-563-1586

Email:- gborthak@mdanderson.org

Study With Azacitidine in Pediatric Subjects With Newly Diagnosed Advanced Myelodysplastic Syndrome (MDS) and Juvenile Myelomonocytic Leukemia (JMML).

Purpose:- Indication Treatment of pediatric subjects with newly diagnosed advanced myelodysplastic syndrome (MDS) or juvenile myelomonocytic leukemia (JMML) prior to hematopoietic stem cell transplantation (HSCT).

Objectives Primary Objective:- The primary objective is to assess the treatment effect on response rate (MDS: either complete remission [CR], partial remission [PR], or marrow CR; JMML: either clinical complete remission [cCR] or clinical partial remission [cPR]); at Cycle 3 Day 28 (each cycle is 28 days) and to compare against standard therapy using a matched-pairs analysis of historical data.

Secondary Objective:- The secondary objective is to further evaluate safety, efficacy, pharmacokinetics (PK), and pharmacodynamics (PD) of azacitidine in this subject population.

Study Design:- This is a prospective, open-label, Phase 2 study consisting of 2 parallel experimental arms, one for each disease group: MDS and JMML. Each arm is designed based on Simon's Optimal 2 stage study design. The sample size has been calculated to allow evaluation of the response rate at 28 day-Cycle 3 Day 28 in each of the 2 disease groups. Each of the experimental arms will also individually be compared against a historical control arm using data retrospectively collected from the European Working Group of MDS in childhood (EWOG-MDS) registry by means of a matched-pairs analysis; matched for predefined subject baseline characteristics defined before any results from this study are known post Stage 1.

Twenty subjects with MDS and 35 JMML subjects evaluable for the primary endpoint (ie, subjects that receive at least 1 dose of investigational product [IP]) will be enrolled at approximately 45 centers in Europe. Each experimental arm has 1 interim analysis planned (at the end of Stage 1). If, during Stage 1 evaluation, less than 2 subjects are observed with a CR, PR, or marrow CR after 3 months of azacitidine in the first 9 subjects with MDS, then enrollment will be stopped. Similarly, if less than 3 subjects are observed with a cPR or cCR after 3 months of azacitidine in the first 18 subjects with JMML, then enrollment will be stopped.

Locations:-

Austria

    St. Anna Kinderkrebsforschung, CHILDREN'S CANCER RESEARCH INSTITUTE
        Vienna, Austria, 1090

Belgium

Hopital Universitaire des Enfants
Brussels, Belgium, 1020

University Hospital Ghent
Ghent, Belgium, 9000

Czech Republic

University Hospital Motol
Prague 5, Czech Republic, 150 06

Denmark

Rigshospitalet
Copenhagen, Denmark, DK-2100

France

Centre Hospitalier Universitaire Lyon
Lyon, France, 69008

Hopital d'Enfants de la Timone
Marseille Cedex 01, France, 13005

Hopital Robert Debre
Paris, France, 75935

Germany

Klinikum Augsburg
Augsburg, Germany, 86156

Charite Berlin
Berlin, Germany, 13353

Universitaetsklinikum Carl Gustav Carus
Dresden, Germany, 01307

Hematology, Oncology and clinical immunology / Heinrich-

Copyright - 2017. Published by Cancer Group Institute. www.cancergroup.com 183

Heine-University
Dusseldorf, Germany, 40225

Universitatsklinikum Essen
Essen, Germany, 45147

Klinikum der Johann Wolfgang Goethe-Universität
Frankfurt/Main
Frankfurt am Main, Germany, 60596

Universitatsklinik
Freiburg, Germany, 79106

University of Hamburg
Hamburg, Germany, 20246

Medizinische Hochschule Hannover
Hannover, Germany, 30625

Universitatsklinikum
Jena, Germany, 7740

Universitatsklinikum Schleswig-Holstein
Kiel, Germany, 24105

Klinikum der Universitaet Muenchen
Munchen, Germany, 80336

Universitatsklinik Munster
Münster, Germany, 48149

Krankenhaus Barmherzige Bruder Regensburg
Regensburg, Germany, 93049

Universitatsklinikum
Tübingen, Germany, 72076

Ireland

Our Lady's Hospital for Sick Children

Copyright - 2017. Published by Cancer Group Institute. www.cancergroup.com 184

Dublin 12, Ireland

Italy

Policlinico Sant'Orsola-Malpighi
Bologna, Italy, 40138

IRCCS Gaslini Hospital
Genova Quarto, Italy, 16148

Azienda Ospedaliera San Gerardo
Monza, Italy, 20900

General Hospital
Padova, Italy, 35128

IRCCS Policlinico San Matteo
Pavia, Italy, 27100

Ospedale Bambin Gesu
Roma, Italy, 00165

Regina Margherita Children's Hospital
Torino, Italy, 10126

Netherlands

Erasmus MC
Rotterdam, Netherlands, 3015 GJ

Spain

Hospital Sant Joan de Deu
Barcelona, Spain, 8950

Hospital Infantil Universitario Nino Jesus
Madrid, Spain, 28009

Hospital Universitario Virgen de La Arrixaca
Murcia, Spain, 30120

Copyright - 2017. Published by Cancer Group Institute. www.cancergroup.com

Sweden

Queen Silvia Childrens Hospital
Gothenburg, Sweden, SE-416 85

Karolinska University Hospital
Stockholm, Sweden, SE-171 76

Switzerland

Universitäts-Kinderklinik
Zurich, Switzerland, 8032

United Kingdom

Great Ormond Street Hospital
London, United Kingdom, WC1N 3JH

Royal Manchester Children's Hospital
Manchester, United Kingdom, M13 9WL

Principal Investigator:- Bouchra Benettaib, MD
Tel:- +1 908-673-9000
Email:- bbenettaib@celgene.com

Beat AML:- Personalized Medicine for Acute Myeloid Leukemia Based on Functional Genomics.

Purpose:- In this study, DNA sequencing, computational biology modeling, and ex vivo drug sensitivity assays will be utilized to define clinically relevant gene mutations and identify potential therapeutics for patients with acute myeloid leukemia (AML).

Primary Outcome Measures:-

- the genomic abnormality spectrum [Time Frame: 5 years]

  AML cells in the peripheral blood and bone marrow samples will be examined by next generation sequencing using an Illumina DNA sequencer. DNA from the skin biopsy will be used as the constitutional reference DNA. Using skin DNA greatly improves the ability to accurately and precisely identify somatic mutations in the AML cells.

- drug sensitivity [Time Frame: 5 years]

  Ex vivo drug sensitivity testing will be performed on each subject's AML cells derived from peripheral blood and bone marrow. AML cell viability will be recorded for each treatment condition after 72 hours of treatment. A rank-ordered list of drugs will be created in order of drug toxicity.

Locations:- United States, Florida
UF Health Cancer Center
Gainesville, Florida, United States, 32608

Principal Investigator:- Barry Sawicki
Tel:- 352-273-9148
Email:- bswcki@ufl.edu

Chart Review Study of Chronic Myelogenous Leukemia (CML) Patients Treated With Imatinib Outside of a Clinical Trial.

Purpose:-

In this study investigators propose to do a chart review of all Chronic Myelogenous Leukemia (CML) patients that are treated outside of a clinical trial with imatinib that come to MDACC for a second opinion. This is an important population of patients that differs in their management from patients treated in clinical trials for several reasons including but not limited to:

1. It represents a very large patient population receiving standard-dose therapy with imatinib. Estimate over 200 patients evaluated and fall in this category.

2. The follow-up for patients in the largest trial using standard-dose imatinib (the IRIS trial, with 553 patients in treated with imatinib) has been limited after the first 12 months. For example, the rate of molecular responses after the first 12 months of therapy was not obtained as samples stopped being collected at that time point.

3. Patients who are or become pregnant during therapy with imatinib have not been eligible for clinical trials with imatinib or had to be taken off study. Thus, there is no information on the effect of imatinib on imatinib on pregnancy and conception, several such patients have been followed at MDACC.

4. This is a patient population that follows therapy mostly as directed by their local oncologists. This is frequently less stringently adhered to the recommended guidelines for imatinib therapy, with more frequent treatment interruptions, and frequently using suboptimal doses of imatinib (i.e., less than 300mg daily). The effect of these treatment interruptions and suboptimal dosing on response and development of resistance is unclear.

Investigators thus plan to conduct a chart review of these patients to study their treatment course before their initial evaluation at MDACC, and between and during visits to MDACC.

Locations:- United States, Texas
University of Texas MD Anderson Cancer Center
Houston, Texas, United States, 77030

Principal Investigator:- Jorge Cortes, M.D.
Tel:- 713-794-5783
Email:- jcortes@mdanderson.org

LY2606368 in Combination With Cytarabine and Fludarabine in Acute Myelogenous Leukemia (AML) and High-Risk Myelodysplastic Syndrome (HRMDS).

Purpose:- The goal of this clinical research study is to study the safety of LY2606368 when given in combination with fludarabine and cytarabine. The effectiveness of the study drug combination when given to patients with relapsed or refractory AML or HRMDS will also be studied.

Primary Outcome Measures:-

- Dose-Limiting Toxicity (DLT) of LY2606368 in Combination With Cytarabine and Fludarabine in Acute Myelogenous Leukemia (AML) and High-Risk Myelodysplastic Syndrome (HRMDS) [Time Frame: 28 days]

  Dose-limiting toxicity (DLT) defined as a clinically significant adverse event or abnormal laboratory value assessed as unrelated to underlying disease, disease progression, intercurrent illness, or concomitant medications and occurring during the first cycle of the trial that meets any of the following criteria:

- CTCAE grade 3 AST (SGOT) or ALT (SGPT) for > 7 days.
- CTCAE grade 4 AST (SGOT) or ALT (SGPT) of any duration.
- All other clinically significant CTCAE grade 3 or 4 toxicities per NCI CTCAE criteria (except for electrolyte disturbances responsive to correction within 24 h, diarrhea, nausea and vomiting that responds to standard medical care).

Locations:- United States, Texas
University of Texas MD Anderson Cancer Center
Houston, Texas, United States, 77030

Principal Investigator:- Gautam Borthakur, MBBS
Tel:- 713-563-1586
Email:- gborthak@mdanderson.org

Scientific Protocol for the Study of Leukemia and Other Hematologic Diseases among Clean-up Workers in Ukraine Following the Chernobyl Accident.

Purpose:-
Leukemia holds a special place in the study of radiation-related cancer because bone marrow is one of the tissues most sensitive to the carcinogenic effect of ionizing radiation, radiogenic leukemia has the shortest latent period among radiation-induced cancers, and its appearance suggests that solid tumors may follow. These same characteristics also contribute to its considerable significance in radiation protection.

There are, nevertheless, important gaps in existing knowledge of radiation-induced leukemia, gaps that derive from characteristics of the study of the atomic bombing of Hiroshima and Nagasaki, and from studies of the effects of medical irradiation and studies of nuclear workers, these being the studies that have provided most of the information to date.

These gaps include the presumed reduction in risk resulting from dose-fractionation and low dose-rate, and the time-response function in the first five years after exposure.

The primary objective of this study is to investigate leukemia risk as a function of such radiation; it would constitute the largest epidemiologic study conducted to date among working-age males, a group of particular concern in establishing occupational radiation safety standards.

In addition, data on cases of multiple myeloma and myelodysplasia identified in the cohort will be collected to test the hypothesis of a dose related association between radiation and increased risk for each of these diseases.

The **primary scientific objectives** of the proposed study are to test the following hypotheses: (a) that there is a dose-related increase in risk of leukemia among these liquidators; (b) that the magnitude of any observed risk per unit dose is less than that seen in the atomic bomb survivors, exposed to essentially instantaneous radiation.

Subsidiary objectives include:- (a) to investigate the nature of the dose-response relationship among liquidators and to identify modifiers of risk, including time since exposure, age at exposure, etc.; (b) to test the hypothesis that there is a dose-related increased risk of multiple myeloma; (c) to test the hypothesis that there is a dose-related increased risk of myelodysplasial; (d) to collect and store buccal cells from about 2,000 liquidators with a wide range of dose estimates extending to well over 1 Gy for possible use in future molecular studies of their DNA.

Primary Outcome Measures:-

- The primary objective of this study is to investigate leukemia risk as a function of radiation ionizing radiation from occupational exposure (Chernobyl nuclear power plant).

Locations:- Ukraine

Research Center for Radiation Medicine

Kiev, Ukraine

Principal Investigator:- Maureen Hatch, M.D.
Tel:- 301-594-7658
Email:- hatchm@mail.nih.gov

Contact:- Kiyohiko Mabuchi, M.D.
Tel:- 301-594-7649
Email:- mabuchik@mail.nih.gov

A Phase I Trial of 4SCAR19 Cells in the Treatment of Relapsed and Refractory B Cell Leukemia.

Purpose:- A chimeric antigen receptor gene-modified T cells (CART: 4SCAR19)by targeted the CD19 (cluster of differentiation antigen 19), treat patients with CD19 positive malignant B cells tumor, assess treatment safety, and observe therapeutic effects. At the same time,the change process of the CART and residual tumor status of the patient are observe dynamically, which summarizes the best therapeutic effect.

Primary Outcome Measures:-

• Safety Using CTCAE 4 standard to evaluate the level of adverse events after receiving the cells. [Time Frame: 24 weeks].

Safety of fourth generation anti CD19 CAR-T cells in patients with relapsed and refractory B-ALL - Using CTCAE 4 standard to evaluate the level of adverse events after receiving the cells.

Locations:- China, Yunnan
First people's hospital of Yunnan province
Kunming, Yunnan, China, NCT650000

Principal Investigator:- Dr. Lai Xun
Tel:- 13577096609
Email:- 1729112214@qq.com

Contact:- Dr. Chang Lung-Ji
b 13671121909
Email:- longflorida@gmail.com

Haploidentical Hematopoietic Stem Cell Transplantation for Acute Leukemias.

Purpose:- This is a prospective observational cohort study of haploidentical transplantation with post-transplant cyclophosphamide for acute leukemias using reduced intensity conditioning for acute myeloid leukemia (AML) and myeloablative conditioning for acute lymphoblastic leukemia (ALL).

Detailed Description:- Hematopoietic stem cell transplantation (HSCT) is the most effective treatment for acute myeloid leukemia (AML) and acute lymphoblastic leukemia (ALL), with the lowest rates of relapse.

Fertility rate in Brazil is falling, and only 25% of people born today will have a matched sibling donor. On the other hand, currently donor non-related to about 50% of patients enrolled in Brazilian Receptor Registry

(REREME). Consequently, at least 35% of patients won't have a matched donor.

The haploidentical transplantation is defined as a partially matched hematopoietic cell transplantation, using a partially matched family donor (parent, sibling or child). Haploidentical transplantation activity is growing worldwide, with results comparable matched unrelated donors.

The objective of this study is to test the feasibility of haploidentical transplantation with post-transplant cyclophosphamide for acute leukemias in a Brazil.

Locations:- Brazil
Instituto Nacional de Cancer
Rio de Janeiro, Brazil, 20230-130

Principal Investigator:- Leonardo J Arcuri, MD
Tel:- +55(21)3207-1304
Email:- leonardojavier@gmail.com

Contact:- Simone Lermontov
Tel:- +55(21)3207-1261
Email:- simonelermontov@globo.com

A Phase II Study of Dasatinib in Children and Adolescents With Newly Diagnosed Chronic Phase CML or With Ph+ Leukemias Resistant or Intolerant to Imatinib.

Purpose:- The purpose of this study is to determine whether dasatinib is safe and effective in children and adolescents with newly diagnosed chronic myeloid leukemia (CML), or in children with Ph+ acute lymphoblastic leukemia (ALL), accelerated or blast phases CML who relapse after imatinib or who are resistant or intolerant to imatinib. The side effects of this oral investigational drug in children and adolescents will be evaluated.

Primary Outcome Measures:-

- Major Cytogenetic Response (MCyR) rate defined as the proportion of all treated subjects who achieve a complete or partial cytogenetic response on study [Time Frame: Up to 5 years].

  MCyR rate will be measured every 3 months during the first two years and yearly thereafter for up to 5 years after discontinuation of study therapy.

- Complete Hematologic Response (CHR) rate defined as the proportion of all treated subjects who achieve a confirmed CHR on study [Time Frame: Up to 5 years].

  CHR rate will be measured every 3 months during the first two years and yearly thereafter for up to 5 years after discontinuation of study therapy

- Complete Cytogenetic Response (CCyR) rate, defined as the proportion of all treated subjects who achieve a CCyR on study [Time Frame: Up to 5 years].

  CCyR rate will be measured every 3 months during the first two years and yearly thereafter for up to 5 years after discontinuation of study therapy.

Locations:-

United States, Arizona

    Phoenix Children'S Hospital

Phoenix, Arizona, United States, 85016

United States, California

Jonathan Jaques Children'S Cancer Center
Long Beach, California, United States, 90806

Children'S Hospital Of Orange County
Orange, California, United States, 92868

United States, Colorado

Children'S Hospital
Aurora, Colorado, United States, 80045

United States, Georgia

Aflac Cancer Center & Blood Disorders Service
Atlanta, Georgia, United States, 30322

United States, Illinois

Children'S Hospital Of Chicago
Chicago, Illinois, United States, 60611

United States, Massachusetts

Dana Faber Cancer Institute
Boston, Massachusetts, United States, 02215

United States, New York

New York University Langone Medical Center
New York, New York, United States, 10016

Memorial Sloan Kettering Cancer Center
New York, New York, United States, 10065

United States, Oregon

Oregon Health & Sci Univ
Portland, Oregon, United States, 97239

United States, Pennsylvania

Children'S Hospital Of Philadelphia
Philadelphia, Pennsylvania, United States, 19104

Children'S Hospital Of Pittsburgh
Pittsburgh, Pennsylvania, United States, 15224

United States, Texas

Md Anderson Cancer Center
Houston, Texas, United States, 77030

Texas Children'S Cancer Center
Houston, Texas, United States, 77030

United States, Washington

Seattle Children'S
Seattle, Washington, United States, 98105

Argentina

Local Institution
Bunos Aires, Buenos Aires, Argentina, 1425

Hospital Nacional Profesor Alejandro Posadas
El Palomar, Buenos Aires, Argentina, 1684

Local Institution
Cordoba, Argentina, 5016

Australia, New South Wales

Local Institution
Randwick, New South Wales, Australia, 2031

Local Institution
Westmead, New South Wales, Australia, 2145

Australia, Queensland

Local Institution
Sth Brisbane, Queensland, Australia, 4101

Australia, South Australia

Local Institution
North Adelaide, South Australia, Australia, 5006

Australia, Victoria

Local Institution
Parkville, Victoria, Australia, 3052

Brazil

Local Institution
Curitiba, Parana, Brazil, 80060

Local Institution
Porto Alegre, Rio Grande Do Sul, Brazil, 90035

Local Institution
Campinas, Brazil, 13083

Local Institution
Sao Paulo, Brazil, 01401

Local Institution
Sao Paulo, Brazil, 04023

Canada, Alberta

Alberta Children'S Hospital
Calgary, Alberta, Canada, T3B 6A8

Stollery Children'S Hospital
Edmonton, Alberta, Canada, T6G 2B7

Canada, British Columbia

Bc Children'S Hospital
Vancouver, British Columbia, Canada, V6H 3V4

Canada, Nova Scotia

Iwk Health Centre
Halifax, Nova Scotia, Canada, B3K 6R8

Canada, Ontario

Children'S Hospital Of Eastern Ontario
Ottawa, Ontario, Canada, K1H 8L1

The Hospital For Sick Children
Toronto, Ontario, Canada, M5G 1X8

Canada, Quebec

Chu Ste-Justine
Montreal, Quebec, Canada, H3T 1C5

France

Local Institution
Lyon, France, 69008

Local Institution
Nantes, France, 44093

Local Institution
Paris Cedex 12, France, 75571

Local Institution
Paris, France, 75935

Local Institution
Poitiers, France, 86000

Germany

Local Institution
Frankfurt, Germany, 60590

Local Institution
Hannover, Germany, 30625

India

Local Institution
Navrangpura, Ahmedabad, Gujarat, India, 380009

Local Institution
Bangalore, Karnataka, India, 560027

Local Institution
Pune, Maharashtra, India, 411001

Local Institution
Madurai, Tamil Nadu, India, 625107

Local Institution
Vellore, Tamilnadu, India, 632004

Local Institution
Kolkatta, India, 700 016

Local Institution
Mumbai, India, 400010

Local Institution
Trivandrum, India, 695011

Italy

Local Institution
Bologna, Italy, 40138

Local Institution
Monza (MB), Italy, 20900

Local Institution
Roma, Italy, 00161

Local Institution
Roma, Italy, 00165

Local Institution
Torino, Italy, 10126

Korea, Republic of

Local Institution
Seoul, Korea, Republic of, 05505

Local Institution
Seoul, Korea, Republic of, 137-701

Mexico

Local Institution
Df, Distrito Federal, Mexico, 06720

Local Institution
Mexico, D. F., Distrito Federal, Mexico, 06726

Local Institution
Mexico, Distrito Federal, Mexico, 04530

Local Institution
Guadalajara, Jalisco, Mexico, 44340

Local Institution
Monterrey, N.l., Nuevo Leon, Mexico, 64180

Local Institution
Monterrey, Nuevo Leon, Mexico, 64460

Netherlands

Local Institution
Rotterdam, Netherlands, 3015 GJ

Romania

Local Institution
Bucharest, Romania, 022322

Russian Federation

Local Institution
Moscow, Russian Federation, 115478

Local Institution
Moscow, Russian Federation, 117198

Local Institution
Saint-petersburg, Russian Federation, 197022

Singapore

Local Institution
Singapore, Singapore, 119228

South Africa

Local Institution

Bloemfontein, Free State, South Africa, 9301

Local Institution
Pretoria, Gauteng, South Africa, 0001

Local Institution
Cape Town, Western Cape, South Africa, 7925

Local Institution
Tygerberg, Western Cape, South Africa, 7505

Spain

Local Institution
Barcelona, Spain, 08025

Local Institution
Barcelona, Spain, 08035

Local Institution
Madrid, Spain, 28009

Local Institution
Madrid, Spain, 28046

Local Institution
Malaga, Spain, 29010

Local Institution
Valencia, Spain

United Kingdom

Local Institution
Glasgow, Central, United Kingdom, G3 8SJ

Local Institution
Sutton, Surrey, United Kingdom, SM2 5PT

Local Institution

A Study Evaluating Venetoclax in Combination With Low-Dose Cytarabine in Treatment-Naïve Subjects With Acute Myelogenous Leukemia (AML).

Purpose:- This study consists of three portions: The first portion- Phase 1, or dose-escalation portion, that will evaluate the safety and pharmacokinetic profile of venetoclax in combination with low-dose cytarabine (LDC), define the maximum tolerated dose (MTD), and generate data to support a recommended Phase 2 dose (RPTD) in treatment-naïve subjects with Acute Myelogenous Leukemia (AML).

Second portion, initial Phase 2 that will evaluate if the RPTD has sufficient efficacy and acceptable toxicity to warrant further development of the combination therapy. Subsequently, Phase 2 Cohort C, will evaluate the overall response rate (ORR) for subjects allowed additional supportive medications (strong CYP3A inhibitors) if medically indicated.

Primary Outcome Measures:

- Number of participants with adverse events [Time Frame: From participant's first dose until 30 days after participant's last dose of study drug; up to 2 years following last participant first dose]

  Participants will be monitored for clinical and laboratory evidence of adverse events throughout the study.

- Maximum observed plasma concentration (Cmax) of venetoclax [Time Frame: Blood samples will be taken at 0 (pre-dose), 2, 4, 6, 8 and 24 hours post-dose on Days 10 and 18.]

  The highest concentration that a drug achieves in the blood after administration in a dosing interval.

- Time to maximum observed plasma concentration (Tmax) of venetoclax [Time Frame: Blood samples will be taken at 0 (pre-dose), 2, 4, 6 ,8 and 24 hours post-dose on Days 10 and 18.]

  The time at which the maximum plasma concentration (Cmax) is observed.

- Area under the plasma concentration-time curve from time 0 to 24 hours post-dose (AUC24) of venetoclax [Time Frame: Blood samples will be taken at 0 (pre-dose), 2, 4, 6, 8, and 24 hours post-dose on Days 10 and 18.]

  The area under the plasma concentration-time curve over a 24-hour dose interval.

- Maximum tolerated dose (MTD) of venetoclax in combination with cytarabine [Time Frame: Minimum first cycle of dosing (28 days)]

  Venetoclax will be dose-escalated until the largest dose is reached that is determined to be safe based on adverse event reporting and dose-limiting toxicity information from all participants.

- Recommended phase two dose (RPTD) of venetoclax in combination with cytarabine [Time Frame: Minimum first cycle of dosing (28 days)]

  Venetoclax will be dose-escalated until the largest dose is reached that is determined to be safe based on adverse event reporting and dose-limiting toxicity information from all participants.

- Overall Response Rate- In Cohort C, overall response rate (ORR) will be evaluated for subjects allowed additional supportive meds

(e.g strong CYP3A inhibitor) if medically indicated.
[Time Frame: Measured up to 2 years after the last participant has enrolled in the study.]

Overall response rate will be defined as the proportion of participants who achieve a complete remission (CR), complete remission with incomplete marrow recovery (CRi), or partial remission (PR) per the International Working Group (IWG) for AML.

- Time to progression (TTP) [Time Frame: Measured up to 2 years after the last participant has enrolled in the study.]

Time to progression will be defined as the number of days from the date of enrollment to the date of earliest disease progression.

- Maximum observed plasma concentration (Cmax) of cytarabine [Time Frame: Blood samples will be taken 0 (pre-dose); 15 and 30 minutes; and 1, 3, and 6 hours after subcutaneous injection on Days 1 and 10.]

The highest concentration that a drug achieves in the blood after administration in a dosing interval

- Time to maximum observed plasma concentration (Tmax) of cytarabine. [Time Frame: Blood samples will be taken 0 (pre-dose); 15 and 30 minutes; and 1, 3, and 6 hours after subcutaneous injection on Days 1 and 10.]

The time at which the maximum plasma concentration (Cmax) is observed.

- Area under the plasma concentration-time curve from time 0 to 6 hours post-dose (AUC6) of cytarabine. [Time Frame: Blood samples will be taken 0 (pre-dose); 15 and 30 minutes; and 1, 3, and 6 hours after subcutaneous injection on Days 1 and 10.]

  The area under the plasma concentration-time curve over a 6-hour dose interval.

- Number of participants with adverse events [Time Frame: From participant's first dose until 30 days after participant's last dose of study drug; up to 2 years following last participant first dose]

  Participants will be monitored for clinical and laboratory evidence of adverse events throughout the study.

- Maximum observed plasma concentration (Cmax) of venetoclax [Time Frame: Blood samples will be taken at 0 (pre-dose), 2, 4, 6, 8 and 24 hours post-dose on Days 10 and 18.]

  The highest concentration that a drug achieves in the blood after administration in a dosing interval.

- Time to maximum observed plasma concentration (Tmax) of venetoclax [Time Frame: Blood samples will be taken at 0 (pre-dose), 2, 4, 6 ,8 and 24 hours post-dose on Days 10 and 18.]

  The time at which the maximum plasma concentration (Cmax) is observed.

- Area under the plasma concentration-time curve from time 0 to 24 hours post-dose (AUC24) of venetoclax [Time Frame: Blood samples will be taken at 0 (pre-dose), 2, 4, 6, 8, and 24 hours post-dose on Days 10 and 18.]

The area under the plasma concentration-time curve over a 24-hour dose interval.

- Maximum tolerated dose (MTD) of venetoclax in combination with cytarabine [Time Frame: Minimum first cycle of dosing (28 days)]

  Venetoclax will be dose-escalated until the largest dose is reached that is determined to be safe based on adverse event reporting and dose-limiting toxicity information from all participants.

- Recommended phase two dose (RPTD) of venetoclax in combination with cytarabine [Time Frame: Minimum first cycle of dosing (28 days)]

  Venetoclax will be dose-escalated until the largest dose is reached that is determined to be safe based on adverse event reporting and dose-limiting toxicity information from all participants.

- Overall Response Rate- In Cohort C, overall response rate (ORR) will be evaluated for subjects allowed additional supportive meds (e.g strong CYP3A inhibitor) if medically indicated.
  [Time Frame: Measured up to 2 years after the last participant has enrolled in the study.]

  Overall response rate will be defined as the proportion of participants who achieve a complete remission (CR), complete remission with incomplete marrow recovery (CRi), or partial remission (PR) per the International Working Group (IWG) for AML.

- Time to progression (TTP) [Time Frame: Measured up to 2 years after the last participant has enrolled in the study.]

Time to progression will be defined as the number of days from the date of enrollment to the date of earliest disease progression.

- Maximum observed plasma concentration (Cmax) of cytarabine [Time Frame: Blood samples will be taken 0 (pre-dose); 15 and 30 minutes; and 1, 3, and 6 hours after subcutaneous injection on Days 1 and 10.]

The highest concentration that a drug achieves in the blood after administration in a dosing interval

- Time to maximum observed plasma concentration (Tmax) of cytarabine. [Time Frame: Blood samples will be taken 0 (pre-dose); 15 and 30 minutes; and 1, 3, and 6 hours after subcutaneous injection on Days 1 and 10.]

The time at which the maximum plasma concentration (Cmax) is observed.

- Area under the plasma concentration-time curve from time 0 to 6 hours post-dose (AUC6) of cytarabine. [Time Frame: Blood samples will be taken 0 (pre-dose); 15 and 30 minutes; and 1, 3, and 6 hours after subcutaneous injection on Days 1 and 10.]

The area under the plasma concentration-time curve over a 6-hour dose interval.

Locations:- United States, New York
New York Presbyterian Hospital /ID# 131170
New York, New York, United States, 10021

United States, Pennsylvania
UPMC Hillman Cancer Center /ID# 131168
Pittsburgh, Pennsylvania, United States, 15232

United States, Tennessee
Vanderbilt University Medical Center /ID# 131177
Nashville, Tennessee, United States, 37232

United States, Washington
Fred Hutchinson Cancer Research Center /ID# 131178
Seattle, Washington, United States, 98109

Australia
The Alfred Hospital /ID# 131180
Melbourne, Australia, 3004

Calvary Mater Newcastle /ID# 136076
Waratah, Australia, 2298

Germany
Universitaetsklinikum Eppendorf Hamburg-CeDeF /ID# 133979
Hamburg, Germany, 20246

Italy
Policlinico Universitario S. Orsola Malpighi /ID# 131183
Bologna, Italy, 40138

Principal Investigator:- John Hayslip, MD
Tel:- 847-283-8955
Email:- abbvieclinicaltrials@abbvie.com

A Novel "Pediatric-Inspired" Regimen With Reduced Myelosuppressive Drugs for Adults (Aged 18-60) With Newly Diagnosed Ph Negative Acute Lymphoblastic Leukemia.

Purpose:- The purpose of the study is to find out whether the combination of chemotherapy drugs that are routinely used in children with ALL, will be safe and effective in treating adult patients with ALL. The standard treatment for adults with ALL consists of many chemotherapy drugs that are given in different combinations and in several steps.

In adult ALL there is no standard which drugs to give and how to combine them. Some leukemias have a chromosome abnormality called Philadelphia chromosome (also called Ph Positive) and some leukemias do not (called Ph Negative).

In this study we want to see whether this combination of chemotherapy drugs will be safe and effective in treating adult patients with Ph Negative ALL.

Primary Outcome Measures:-
- rate of molecular remission [Time Frame: 1 year].

    i.e. minimal residual disease (MRD) negative status, as assessed by PCR and flow cytometry in the bone marrow after phase I induction.

Locations:- United States, New York

Memorial Sloan Kettering Cancer Center

New York, New York, United States, 10065

Contact:- Jae Park, MD

Contact:- Martin Tallman, MD

Tel:- 212-639-4048

Email:- tallmanm@mskcc.org

Weill Cornell Medical Center   Recruiting
New York, New York, United States
Contact:- Ellen Ritchie, MD
Principal Investigator:- Ellen Ritchie, MD

United States, North Carolina
Duke University Medical Center
Durham, North Carolina, United States, 27701

United States, Pennsylvania
Lehigh Valley Health Network
Allentown, Pennsylvania, United States, 18103
Contact:- Brian Patson, MD
Tel:- 610-402-7880

Principal Investigator:- Jae Park, MD
Tel:- 212-639-4048
Email:- Parkj6@mskcc.org

A Phase II Study of Ibrutinib Plus FCR in Previously Untreated, Younger Patients With Chronic Lymphocytic Leukemia (iFCR).

Purpose:- This research study is evaluating a new drug called ibrutinib in combination with the standard drugs fludarabine, cyclophosphamide, and rituximab (FCR) as a possible treatment for Chronic Lymphocytic Leukemia (CLL).

Copyright - 2017. Published by Cancer Group Institute. www.cancergroup.com

Primary Outcome Measures:- Rate of MRD Negative Complete Response [Time Frame: 2 months after completing combination therapy]. Clopper-Pearson binomial method.

Locations:- United States, Maine

Eastern Maine Medical Center

Brewer, Maine, United States, 04412

Contact:- Laurie Lewis

Email:- llewis@emhs.org

United States, Massachusetts

Massachusetts General Hospital

Boston, Massachusetts, United States, 02114

Contact: Jeremy Abramson, MD

Principal Investigator:- Jeremy Abramson, MD

Tel:- 617-726-8743

Email:- jabramson@partners.org

Dana Farber Cancer Institute

Boston, Massachusetts, United States, 02215

Contact: Matthew Davids, MD

Principal Investigator:- Matthew Davids, MD

Tel:- 617-632-5847

Email:- matthew_davids@dfci.harvard.edu

United States, Michigan

West Michigan Cancer Center

Kalamazoo, Michigan, United States, 49007

Contact:- Don Park, MD

Email:- dpark@wmcc.org

Contact:- Joan Westendorp

Email:- jwestendorp@wmcc.org

United States, North Carolina

Duke University Medical Center
Durham, North Carolina, United States, 27710

Bosutinib Dose-Optimization Study in Chronic Myeloid Leukemia (CML).

Purpose:- Bosutinib is a type of tyrosine kinase inhibitor (TKI) which is commonly used for the treatment of chronic phase chronic myelogenous leukemia (CP CML). The standard dose of bosutinib often causes temporary, but severe, diarrhea which goes away after bosutinib is stopped or the dose is lowered.

The goal of this clinical research study it to learn if a lower dose of bosutinib is as effective as the standard dose. Researchers think that by starting with a lower dose of bosutinib and slowly increasing the dose (if needed), the likelihood and severity of diarrhea and other side effects may be lowered in patients with CP CML.

Copyright - 2017. Published by Cancer Group Institute. www.cancergroup.com 214

To help researchers learn if the lower dose of bosutinib is as effective as the regular dose, researchers will test your cytogenetic response to the drug. Cytogenetic testing looks at how genetic changes to cells (in this study, the BRC-ABL protein and Philadelphia chromosome) may affect how the disease may react to the study drug.

Primary Outcome Measures:-

- Major Cytogenetic Response Rate of Bosutinib in Participants with Chronic Phase Chronic Myeloid Leukemia Who Have Experienced Resistance or Intolerance to Frontline Tyrosine Kinase Inhibitor Therapy [Time Frame: 6 months]

  Cytogenetic assessments based on at least 20 metaphases or fluorescence in situ hybridization with at least 200 cells on peripheral blood or bone marrow (if cytogenetics are not available).

Locations:- United States, Texas
University of Texas MD Anderson Cancer Center
Houston, Texas, United States, 77030

Principal Investigator:- Philip A. Thompson, MBBS
Tel:- 713-792-7430
Email:- pathompson2@mdanderson.org

There is a bright future for patients who make choices for bettering their health and gaining complete healing through natural and alternative therapies. It is our greatest hope that you will have the confidence using this publication as a guideline that these alternatives are the way to heal your body.

If you wish to have 6 months free of updates on breast cancer. Send an e-mail to cancergroup@gmail.com along with your order number.

Copyright - 2017. Published by Cancer Group Institute. www.cancergroup.com

www.ingramcontent.com/pod-product-compliance
Lightning Source LLC
Chambersburg PA
CBHW061436180526
45170CB00004B/1434

* 9 7 8 1 5 4 6 8 5 6 2 4 5 *